W0018312

ALLERGIC DISORDERS

Allergic Disorders

Edited by

William F Jackson

MA MB BChir MRCP

Formerly Honorary Consultant in Allergy
Department of Medicine, Guy's Hospital
London, England

Mosby-Wolfe

Chicago London Philadelphia St. Louis Sydney Tokyo

Acknowledgements

The editor and contributors gratefully acknowledge the help of a number of individuals who allowed the use of their illustrations in this title:

J.O. Warner, Southampton, UK, **1.11, 1.12, 3.8, 3.9, 3.18, 3.22**; P. Fireman, Pittsburgh, Pennsylvania, US, **1.17, 5.11**; S.J. Challacombe, London, UK, **2.23**; G.M. Cochrane, London, UK, **2.30**; R. Dinwiddie, London, UK, **3.6, 3.11, 3.12, 3.19**; C. O'Callaghan, Leicester, UK, **3.20**.

Project Manager:	Moira Sarsfield
Desk Editor:	Stephen McGrath
Layout:	Marie McNestry
Cover design:	Pete Wilder
Illustration:	Richard Prime
Production:	Mell Van de Velde Mary Sketch
Index:	Anne McCarthy

Published in 1997 by Mosby-Wolfe, an imprint of Times Mirror International Publishers Ltd., Lynton House, 7–12 Tavistock Square, London WC1H 9LB, England, UK. Tel: +44 (0) 171 388 7676; Fax: +44 (0) 171 391 6558.

Printed by Grafos S.A. Arte Sobre Papel, Barcelona, Spain.

Contents

Contributors

Rino Cerio BSc FRCP (Edin) FRCP (London) DipRCPath
Consultant Dermatologist
The Royal London and St Bartholomew's Hospitals, London, UK

Ronald Dahl MD
Professor, Department of Respiratory Diseases
University Hospital of Århus, Århus, Denmark

William F Jackson MA MB BChir MRCP
Formerly Honorary Consultant in Allergy
Department of Medicine, Guy's Hospital, London, England

Anthony D Milner MD FRCP DCH
Consultant Paediatrician, Guy's and St Thomas' Hospital Trust
Professor of Paediatrics and Chairman of Division,
United Medical and Dental Schools of Guy's and St Thomas', London, UK

Niels Mygind MD
Associate Professor, Department of Respiratory Diseases
University Hospital of Århus, Århus, Denmark

Michael G Pearson MA MB BChir FRCP
Consultant Physician, Aintree Chest Centre
Fazakerley Hospital, Liverpool, UK

Michael J Radcliffe MB ChB MRCGP FAAEM
General Practitioner, Southampton, UK
Honorary Consultant Allergist, The Middlesex Hospital, London, UK

P John Rees MD FRCP
Consultant Physician, Guy's and St Thomas' Hospital Trust
Senior Lecturer in Medicine
United Medical and Dental Schools of Guy's and St Thomas', London, UK

Lawrence Youlten MB BS PhD FRCP(Edin) FFPharmMed
Consultant in Applied Pharmacology, Department of Allergy and Respiratory Medicine
Guy's and St Thomas' Hospital Trust, London, UK

Preface

Allergic disorders are common, affecting 15–20% of the population in most developed countries. Up to 30% of the population are atopic, as indicated by positive skin prick tests to one or more common allergens, so the potential for allergic disorders is even greater than their current population prevalence. In addition, the prevalence of allergic disorders has increased over the past 20–30 years. Although the reasons for this increase are unclear, it seems likely that interactions between heredity and environment are pivotal in the development of allergic disorders, and that the critical interactions may occur in infancy, or even during fetal life.

In the long-term, the management of allergic disorders may include their prevention by effective intervention during early life. At present, however, they must usually be diagnosed and treated in their developed state, and this book aims to outline the ideal diagnosis and management of the common allergic disorders.

At first sight, the disorders included in this book could seem a disparate group of conditions, but there are many similarities in their underlying mechanisms. In Chapter 1, Niels Mygind and Ronald Dahl outline key mechanisms in allergic rhinitis, and many of these are equally relevant to other allergic disorders. For example, many allergic disorders involve both immediate symptoms, induced by mediators released in response to allergen exposure, and later (often prolonged) symptoms associated with inflammation of the affected tissue. Correspondingly, the management of allergic disorders often involves inhibition or blockade of mediator action (as by antihistamines and beta-agonists) and suppression of inflammation (usually by corticosteroids).

Each chapter of the book includes a fold-out algorithm summarising the overall management of the condition, and the aim of all contributors has been to give a practical summary, which should be of use to a broad range of readers. These summaries are accompanied by a wide range of useful photographs, tables and diagrams, and by more specialised algorithms where these are appropriate.

Many of the photographs were supplied by the contributors, but others throughout the book come from my own collection and from other colleagues, including contributors to other chapters of the book. I am grateful to all colleagues, photographers and patients who have allowed me to use these photographs now and in the past. A list of those who have granted permission specifically for this book appears elsewhere.

I am very grateful to all the contributors for their speedily produced contributions and for their rapid and full cooperation during editing. I am also particularly grateful to Moira Sarsfield for coordinating the entire project, to Stephen McGrath for his major input to the editing process and to Marie McNestry and Richard Prime for their excellent work on design, illustration and layout, which undoubtedly enhances the educational value of the book.

William F. Jackson
Harwell, Oxford, UK

Allergic inflammation

The clinical features of allergic rhinitis are associated with inflammation of the nasal mucous membrane. The inflammatory process involves infiltration by immune cells, including mast cells, eosinophils, and T lymphocytes, and the release of cytokines and inflammatory mediators, including histamine, leukotrienes and prostaglandins (**Fig. 1.7**). The recruitment of immune cells from the blood to the nasal mucosa is regulated by adhesion molecules such as intercellular adhesion molecule-1 (ICAM-1).

Histamine released from mast cells stimulates sensory nerves and induces reflex-mediated sneezing and hypersecretion. By a direct effect on vascular histamine receptors, it also causes vasodilatation and oedema formation (**Fig. 1.8**). The clinical effect of antihistamines in allergic rhinitis indicates that the principal effects of histamine are to produce sneezing and watery hypersecretion. Histamine is less important in nasal blockage, which is mediated by leukotrienes, and plays no part in the development of nasal hyper-

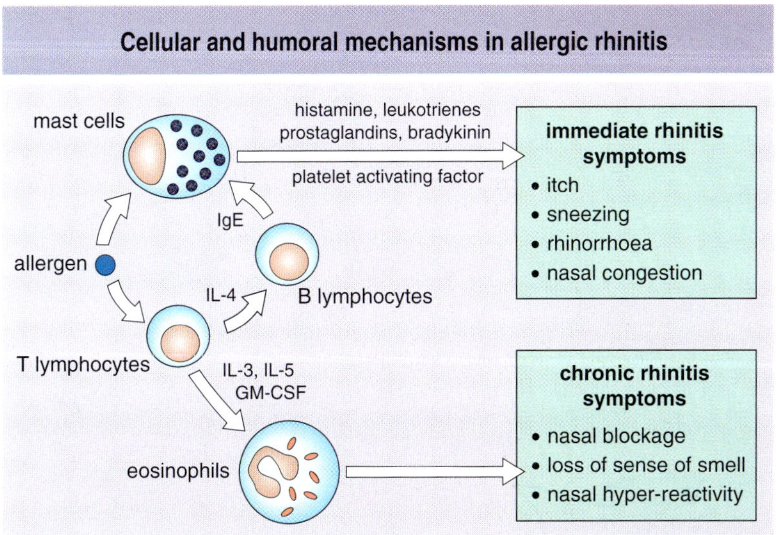

Cellular and humoral mechanisms in allergic rhinitis

mast cells
histamine, leukotrienes prostaglandins, bradykinin
platelet activating factor
IgE
allergen
IL-4
B lymphocytes
T lymphocytes
IL-3, IL-5 GM-CSF
eosinophils

immediate rhinitis symptoms
- itch
- sneezing
- rhinorrhoea
- nasal congestion

chronic rhinitis symptoms
- nasal blockage
- loss of sense of smell
- nasal hyper-reactivity

Fig. 1.7 Cellular and humoral mechanisms in allergic rhinitis. The recruitment of immune cells from the blood to the nasal mucosa is regulated by adhesion molecules such as intercellular adhesion molecule-1 (ICAM-1). T lymphocytes play an important role in orchestrating the inflammatory response, by their release of cytokines, including interleukins (IL) and granulocyte-macrophage colony stimulating factor (GM-CSF). Mast cells play an important role in immediate symptoms, via the release of histamine and other mediators, while eosinophils contribute substantially to the chronic features of rhinitis.

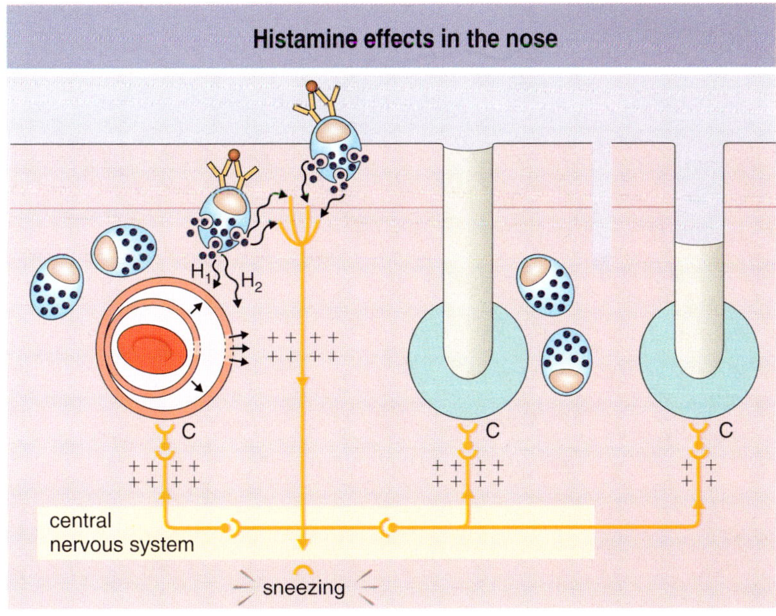

Fig. 1.8 Histamine effects in the nose. Histamine acts directly on vascular histamine receptors causing vasodilatation (H_1 and H_2 receptors), plasma exudation and oedema formation (H_1 receptors). Histamine stimulates sensory nerves (H_1 receptors) and initiates a parasympathetic reflex via cholinoceptors (C), which results in hypersecretion in both sides of the nose. From: Mygind N. Mediators of nasal allergy. *J Allergy Clin Immunol* 1982;**70**:149–59.

responsiveness, which is mediated by eosinophil proteins (**Fig. 1.9**).

The nervous system

The sensory nerves in the nose are more exposed to stimulation from cold, dry and polluted ambient inhaled air than are the bronchial nerves, and there is a constant reflex activity in the nose which stimulates glandular secretion, and modulates vascular tone and nasal patency. Thus, mild symptoms can often be considered as an expression of normal nasal physiology.

Hyper-responsiveness

Both allergic and non-allergic rhinitis are characterized by increased reflex activity and a hyper-responsive mucous membrane. The symptoms of rhinitis can then appear following exposure to a variety of non-specific, everyday stimuli (e.g. cold air, dust, fumes, paint, printing ink, polluted air, washing powder, hot spicy food or alcoholic beverages).

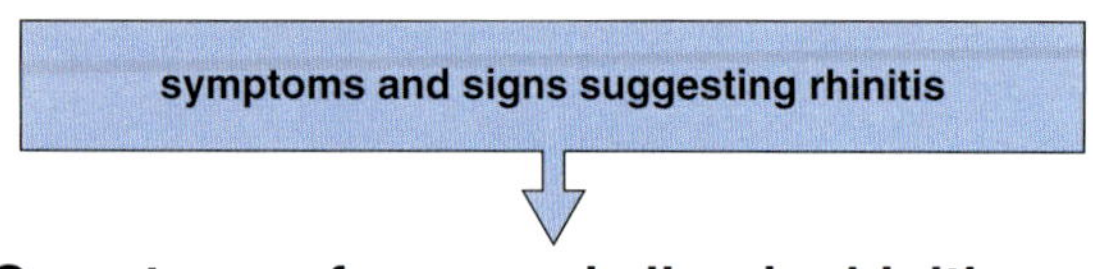

Symptoms of seasonal allergic rhinitis

Itching in the nose results in serial sneezing and watery rhinorrhoea. There can be itching in the throat and referred itching in the ears (**Fig. 1.10**). Congestion in the nose is usually mild or moderate. Itching of the eyes leads to eye rubbing, and a vicious circle is started which can cause red and smarting eyes.

Some patients, especially those with severe allergy, develop bronchial symptoms at the peak of the pollen season. Patients with seasonal allergic rhinitis often have bronchial hyper-responsiveness all year round. If they are sensitized to perennial allergens, they have an increased risk of developing perennial asthma. The severity of eye and nose symptoms varies with the daily pollen count, while the correlation is less obvious for asthma. The pollen count is usually high in sunny, dry weather and low in cold, rainy periods.

In childhood and adolescence, seasonal rhinitis may lead to under-performance in school examinations, which are commonly held at the height of the grass pollen season. The effects of the rhinitis may be exacerbated if sedating antihistamines are used in its treatment.

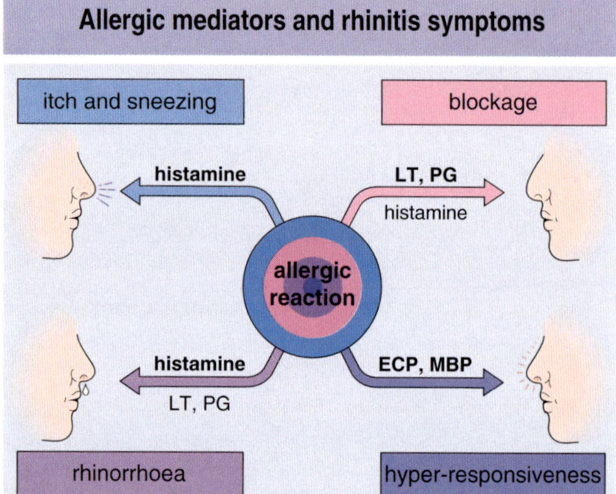

Fig. 1.9 Allergic mediators and rhinitis symptoms. The allergic reaction in the nasal mucous membrane results in release of mediators which, in various combinations, are responsible for the symptoms of allergic rhinitis (LT, leukotrienes; PG, prostaglandins; ECP, eosinophil cationic protein; MBP, major basic protein).

Symptom profile in allergic rhinitis

	Seasonal	Perennial
Sneezing	+++	+
Rhinorrhoea	++	++
Nasal blockage	+	+++
Eye itch	+++	+
Mouth itch	++	–
Asthma	+	++

Fig. 1.10 Symptom profile in allergic rhinitis.

Symptoms of perennial allergic rhinitis

Symptoms are largely the same as those of hay fever, but eye itching is less frequent and nasal blockage more prominent. The average number of sneezes, number of nose blowings and daily duration of symptoms are useful measures of severity.

In children, rhinitis may lead to chronic sniffing and rhinorrhoea, which can be a cause of discord between parent or schoolteacher, and the child. Nevertheless, children's nasal symptoms are often ignored, and allergic rhinitis is under-diagnosed. This is unfortunate, as simple and effective treatment is usually possible.

Many patients, children in particular, also suffer from atopic eczema or asthma. A persistent cough or wheeziness following exercise suggests the co-existence of mild asthma.

Signs

The face often shows characteristic signs in children with perennial allergic rhinitis. If nasal obstruction is severe, an open-mouthed face is seen, which can predispose the child to a high-arched palate, overbite and dental malocclusion (**Fig. 1.11**). Children with allergic rhinitis often develop characteristic mannerisms related to nasal itching (**Fig. 1.12**). Repeated upwards rubbing of the nose – the 'allergic salute' (**Fig. 1.13**) – is common, and

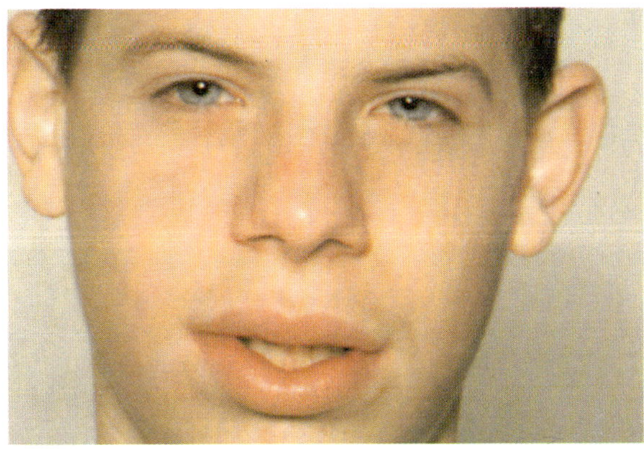

Fig. 1.11 Nasal signs in chronic perennial rhinitis. This 14-year-old boy is allergic to house dust mite, and has had symptoms of rhinitis since early childhood. Note the broadening of the bridge of the nose – and the oedema and slight reddening of the infra-orbital areas. This patient also has mild atopic eczema and episodes of urticaria and angioedema.

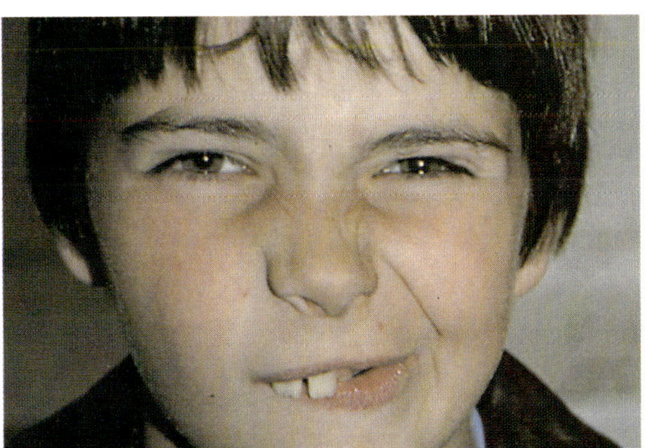

Fig. 1.12 Facial twitching or grimacing is a common accompaniment to allergic rhinitis, and may help to relieve the itching associated with the condition.

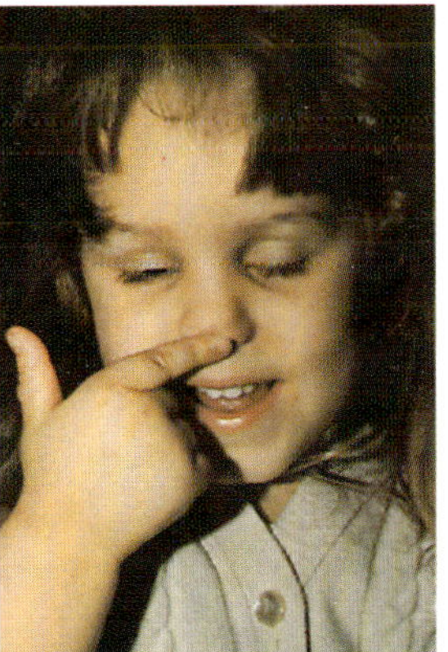

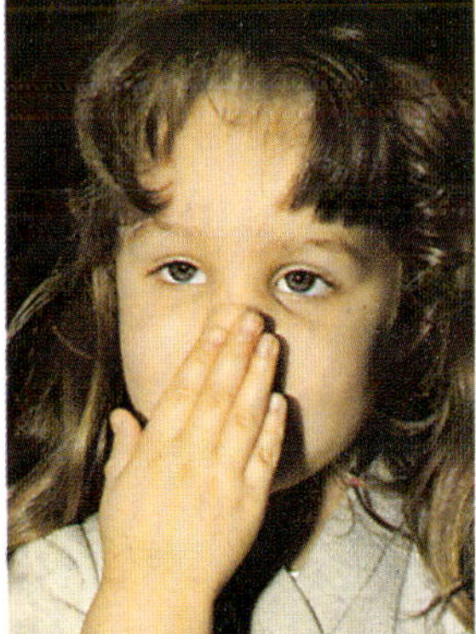

Fig. 1.13 The characteristic facial appearance of a child with allergic rhinitis. This little girl has chronic rhinitis, shown by her habit of rubbing her nose to relieve itching, and by the characteristic allergic salute, in which the fingers and palm of the hand are rubbed upwards over the tip of the nose.

eventually results in the development of a transverse nasal crease (**Fig. 1.14**). Dark rings and congested skin folds (Dennie–Morgan infraorbital folds) (**Fig. 1.15**) are often seen below the eyes in nasal allergy.

exclude physical abnormalities and other diseases

In making the diagnosis, other diseases and structural abnormalities must be excluded (**Fig. 1.16**). Where a posteriorly placed foreign body (**Fig. 1.17**) or an anatomical abnormality such as partial choanal atresia is a possibility, further examination, for example with a fibreoptic endoscope or by contrast radiography, may be required. Enlarged adenoids are not caused by allergic rhinitis, but they may confound the problem of nasal obstruction. They are best demonstrated in young children by X-ray examination of the post-nasal space (**Fig. 1.18**).

Rhinoscopy is indicated in all patients with chronic nasal symptoms. While examination with a speculum and mirror provides limited information, a flexible or rigid endoscope is an excellent tool for the precise diagnosis of anatomical abnormalities, nasal polyps and

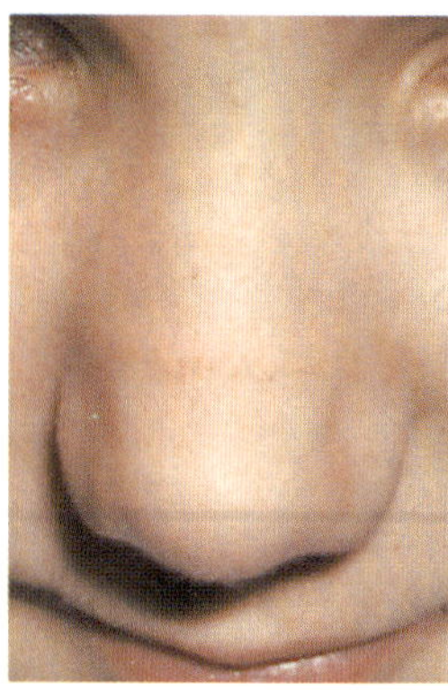

Fig. 1.14 A transverse nasal crease resulting from the allergic salute. This 10-year-old girl with perennial rhinitis had been rubbing her nose upwards with the palm of her hand regularly for several years. Note the oedematous enlargement of the bridge of her nose and upper cheeks, a sign commonly associated with chronic rhinitis.

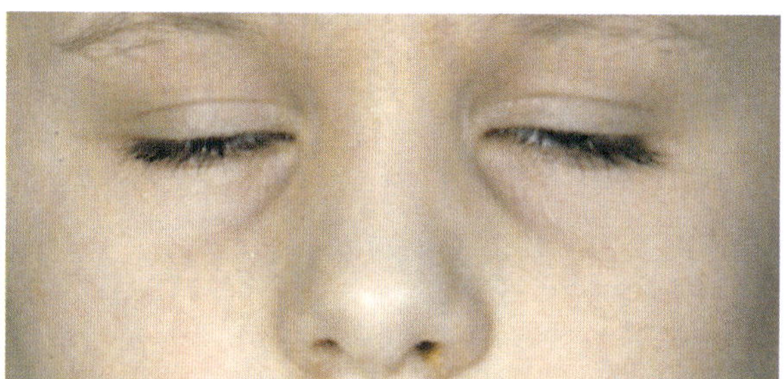

Fig. 1.15 Dennie–Morgan infra-orbital folds. This 10-year-old boy had allergic rhinitis, allergic conjunctivitis, and atopic eczema.

Differential diagnosis of allergic rhinitis

Mechanical factors	Infections	Miscellaneous
Septal deviation	Viral infection (common cold)	Rhinitis medicamentosa
Abnormal ostiomeatal complex	Bacterial infection	Cocaine abuse
Nasal polyps	Sinusitis	Pregnancy
Foreign body	Leprosy	Antihypertensive drugs
Tumours of the nose and sinuses	Immunodeficiency	Wegener's granulomatosis
Tumours of the nasopharynx	Primary ciliary dyskinesia	Cystic fibrosis
Congenital choanal atresia		
Meningocele/encephalocele		Leak of cerebrospinal fluid
Adenoidal hypertrophy		

Fig. 1.16 Differential diagnosis of allergic rhinitis.

sinusitis, and for the exclusion of differential diagnoses. A swollen, wet, pale-blue mucous membrane supports a diagnosis of rhinitis (**Fig. 1.19**).

A *CT scan* of the nose and paranasal sinuses is indicated in selected patients, and is the examination of choice (i) in chronic severe rhinitis, (ii) for excluding malignancy, and (iii) in planning intranasal and sinus surgery (**Fig. 1.20**).

Microscopy of a nasal smear can be helpful in distinguishing between infectious and non-infectious rhinitis, and between eosinophilic rhinitis (allergic and non-allergic) and non-eosinophilic rhinitis. A wiped smear can be obtained using a tightly wound cotton swab. Better specimens and more reproducible results can be obtained with a curette or a cytology brush. When a rapid staining method is used the specimen is ready for mi-

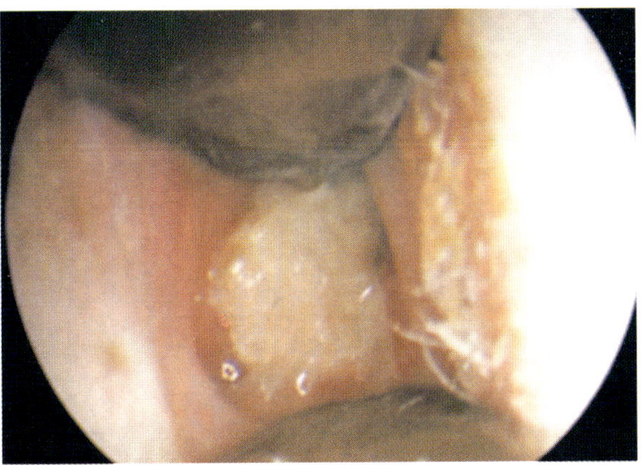

Fig. 1.17 An impacted foreign body in the nose is a commonly overlooked differential diagnosis in suspected allergic rhinitis. Rhinoscopy with a conventional speculum or a fibreoptic endoscope is essential. This child had pushed a piece of plastic foam into his nose.

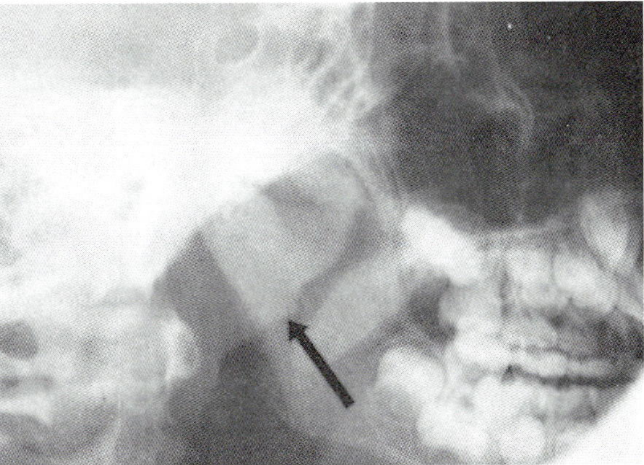

Fig. 1.18 Adenoidal enlargement. The post-nasal space is often very difficult to see on conventional examination in children, and a lateral radiograph may be helpful. Here the airway is almost completely occluded by a large adenoidal pad (arrow). Adenoidal enlargement is common in both atopic and non-atopic children, but it may compound the problem of nasal obstruction in children with allergic rhinitis.

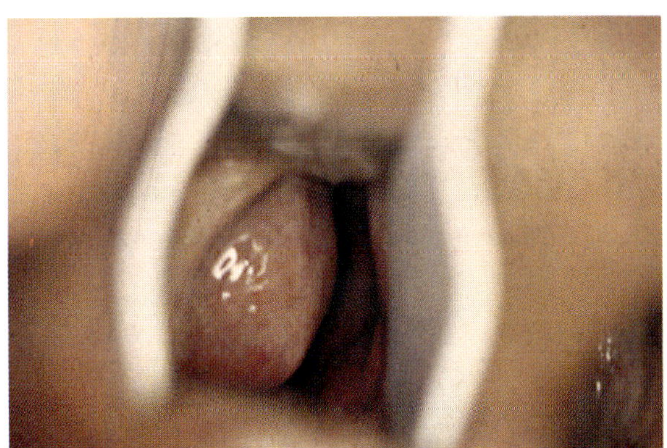

Fig. 1.19 Rhinoscopy. In perennial rhinitis, allergic as well as non-allergic, the mucous membrane of the inferior turbinate is typically swollen, wet, and pale-blue in colour.

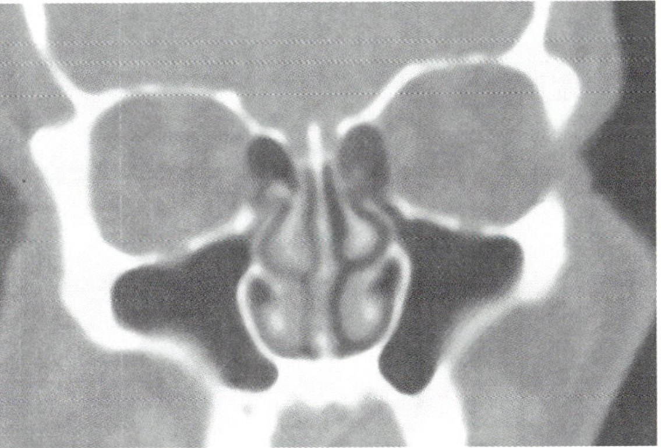

Fig. 1.20 CT scan of the nose and paranasal sinuses gives an excellent presentation of the anatomy. Note how the mucous membrane in the nose takes the shape of the surrounding structures, creating a slit-like air passage.

croscopy within minutes. Eosinophilia (more than 10% eosinophils) is suggestive of either allergic rhinitis or non-allergic eosinophilic rhinitis (**Fig. 1.21**).

skin prick testing

Allergy testing is indicated in severe cases of hay fever, and in all patients with chronic rhinitis. *Skin prick testing* is clinically the most useful allergy test (**Fig. 1.22**). It is simple, quick, and virtually painless, with a high degree of specificity and an extremely low risk of anaphylactic reaction. A prick test wheal of 3 mm or larger is immunologically specific, provided the control test with the diluent is negative (**Fig. 1.23**).

A positive skin test for aero-allergen correlates well with the appearance of allergen-induced symptoms. Thus, a positive pollen test can occur in a symptom-free subject, but indicates a 10-fold increase in the risk of developing of hay fever. This link is weaker for food allergens. Only a fraction of patients with positive tests will react during a food challenge, so false positive reactions are frequent.

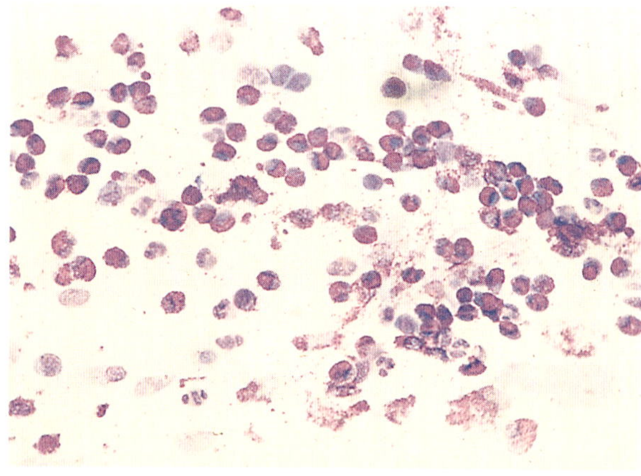

Fig. 1.21 Eosinophilia in a nasal smear as seen in allergic rhinitis, perennial non-allergic eosinophilic rhinitis, and nasal polyposis.

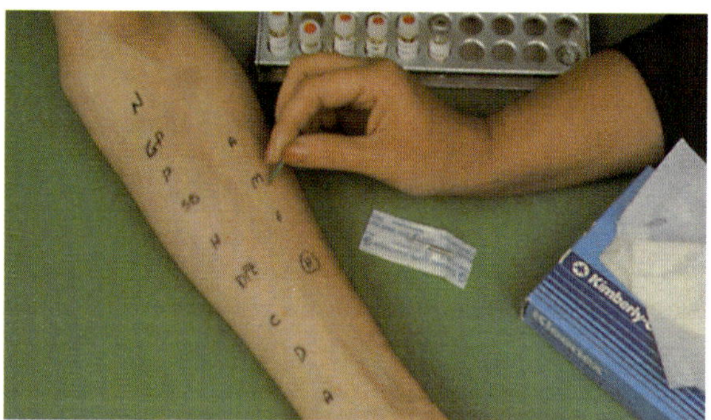

Fig. 1.22 Skin prick testing. A drop of allergen extract is placed on the skin, which is punctured by a 1 mm lancet. This test should always include a negative control of the diluent, since patients with sensitive and dermographic skin can react to the trauma itself. A positive control with histamine allows the clinician to judge the reactivity of the skin and to detect interfering antihistamine medication. Antihistamines depress skin reactivity considerably and treatment must be discontinued before testing (4 days are sufficient for most preparations but 4 weeks are needed for astemizole). The precision of the test can be improved if it is done in duplicate.

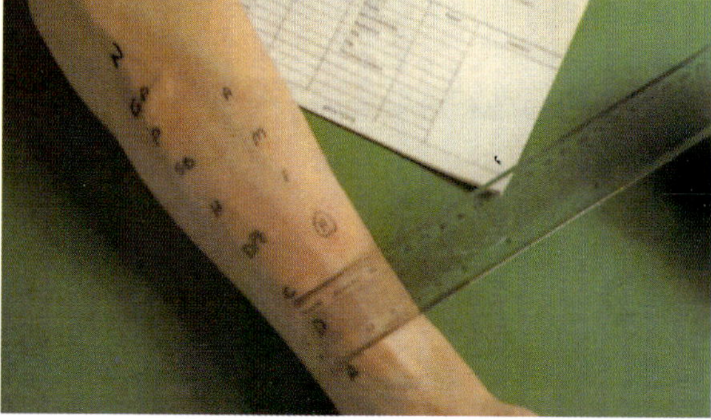

Fig. 1.23 Reading the skin prick test result. A positive weal-and-flare (oedema and erythema) reaction is suggested by itching and erythema and confirmed by the typical mosquito bite-like, flat elevation (weal) which is both seen and felt. It is maximal after 15 minutes. To obtain a permanent record the weal reaction can be outlined by a felt-tip pen and the markings transferred to squared paper by means of tape.

Radioallergosorbent testing (RAST) detects allergen-specific IgE antibody in serum. RAST is well tolerated, shows a high degree of precision and standardization, and is not affected by skin reactivity or concomitant medication. Disadvantages include its high cost, and the fact that results are not immediately available.

allergen avoidance

This is the first measure to be recommended in allergic airway disease, but is not always practicable.

For patients suffering from hay fever, some exposure to pollen is inevitable, since allergen avoidance in the open air is clearly not possible. Even so, excessive exposure can usually be avoided if common sense is applied.

Measures to reduce the population of house mites often have disappointing results, unless radical changes are made (e.g. removing all curtains, carpets and soft furnishings). However, changes in the patient's bedroom can be effective in reducing the allergen burden (**Fig. 1.24**). Improved ventilation and reduced humidity probably provide the best long-term solution to the problem, but may reduce the energy-efficiency of the house unless costly heat-exchanging equipment is also fitted.

Avoidance of pets is easy, but their allergens may linger in a house long after they have gone. Thus it may be some months before the full benefit of an animal's removal is felt. Indirect exposure from animal protein in others' clothes can not be avoided.

House dust mite control measures in the bedroom
The bedroom should be for the sole use of the patient
Keep the room free of animals, tobacco smoke, and unnecessary items that might collect dust
The room floor should be of vinyl, linoleum or wood, so that it is smooth and easy to clean
Avoid all unnecessary items that might collect dust
Only allow simple furniture and washable curtains
Buy a new mattress and encase it in an allergen-impermeable cover
Replace old feather pillows with new foam pillows; then encase them or wash them regularly
Replace old quilts with new ones and wash regularly (>55°C or 130°F)
Replace old eiderdowns with new ones and encase them
Clean, vacuum and change bed linen regularly

Fig. 1.24 House-dust mite control measures in the bedroom.

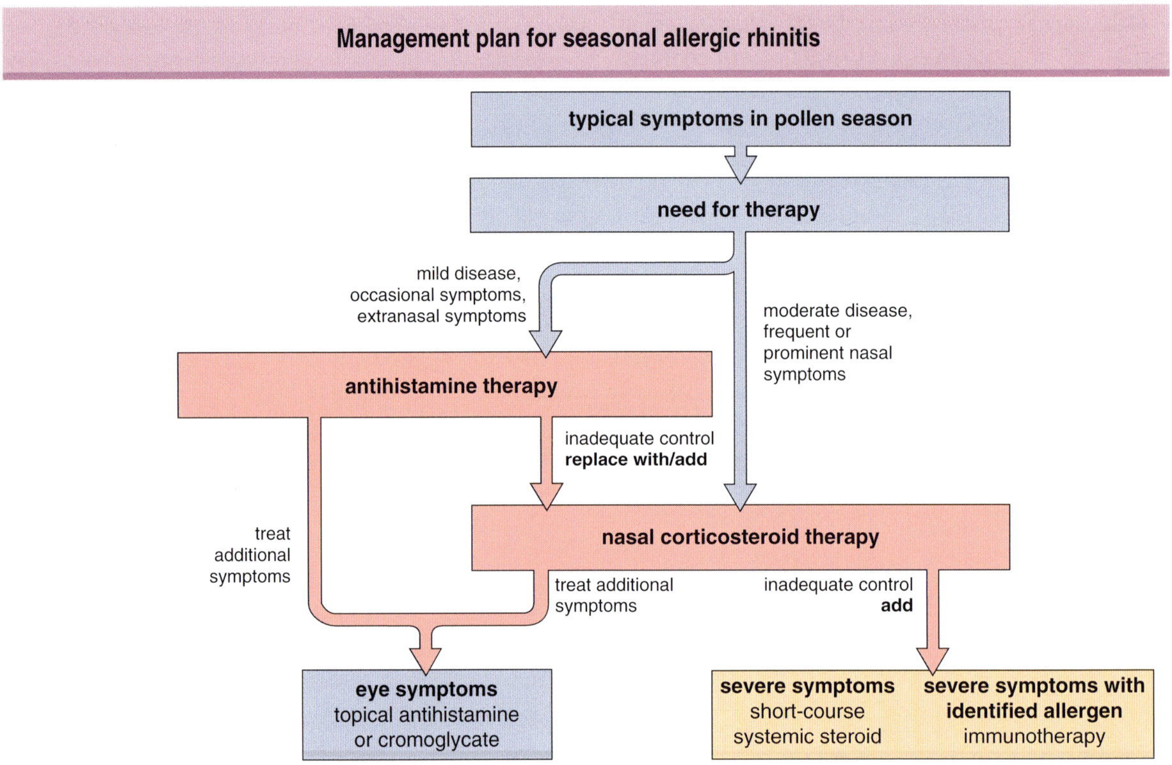

Management plan for seasonal allergic rhinitis
typical symptoms in pollen season
need for therapy
mild disease, occasional symptoms, extranasal symptoms
moderate disease, frequent or prominent nasal symptoms
antihistamine therapy
inadequate control
replace with/add
treat additional symptoms
nasal corticosteroid therapy
treat additional symptoms
inadequate control
add
eye symptoms
topical antihistamine or cromoglycate
severe symptoms
short-course systemic steroid
severe symptoms with identified allergen
immunotherapy

Fig. 1.25 Management plan for seasonal allergic rhinitis.

Management plan for perennial allergic rhinitis in adults
need for therapy
mild disease, occasional symptoms, extranasal symptoms
moderate disease, frequent or prominent nasal symptoms
antihistamine therapy (oral or nasal)
inadequate control
replace with/add
treat additional symptoms
nasal corticosteroid therapy
treat additional symptoms
inadequate control
add
eye symptoms
topical antihistamine or cromoglycate
nasal blockage
nasal decongestion
rhinorrhoea
ipratropium bromide
severe symptoms
short-course systemic steroid

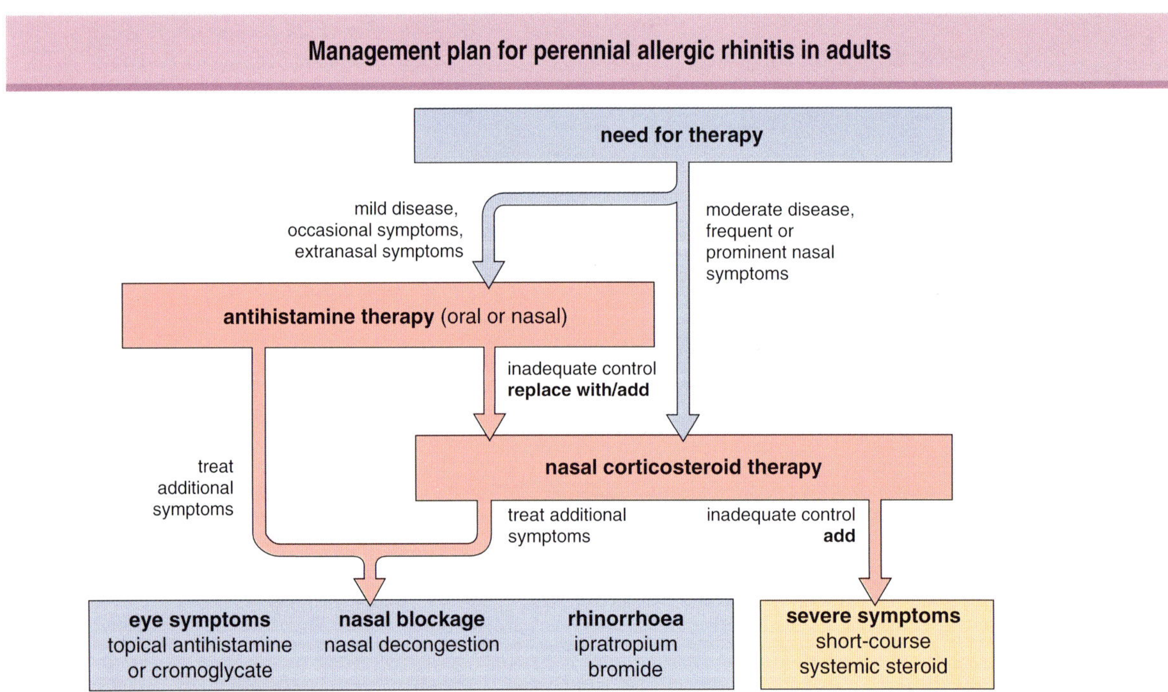

Fig. 1.26 Management plan for perennial allergic rhinitis in adults.

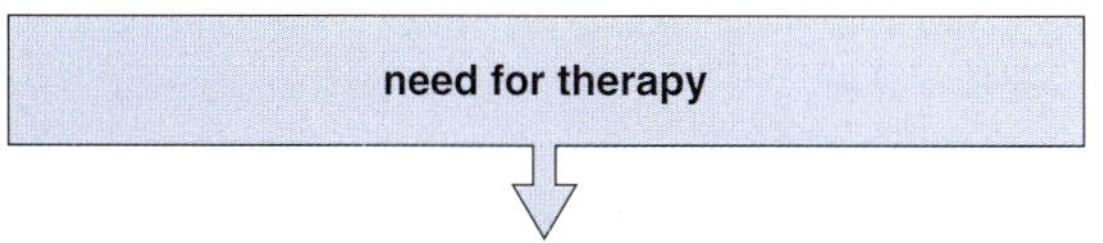

All patients with seasonal and perennial allergic rhinitis, and most patients with perennial non-allergic rhinitis, benefit from drug therapy (**Figs 1.25–1.27**). This should be carefully selected on the basis of the patient's symptomatology (**Fig. 1.28**). Antihistamines are highly effective against the IgE- and mast cell-mediated acute symptoms of rhinitis, including nasal itch, sneezing, and rhinorrhoea. Anti-inflammatory therapy is necessary to counteract chronic symptoms such as nasal blockage, anosmia and nasal hyper-responsiveness.

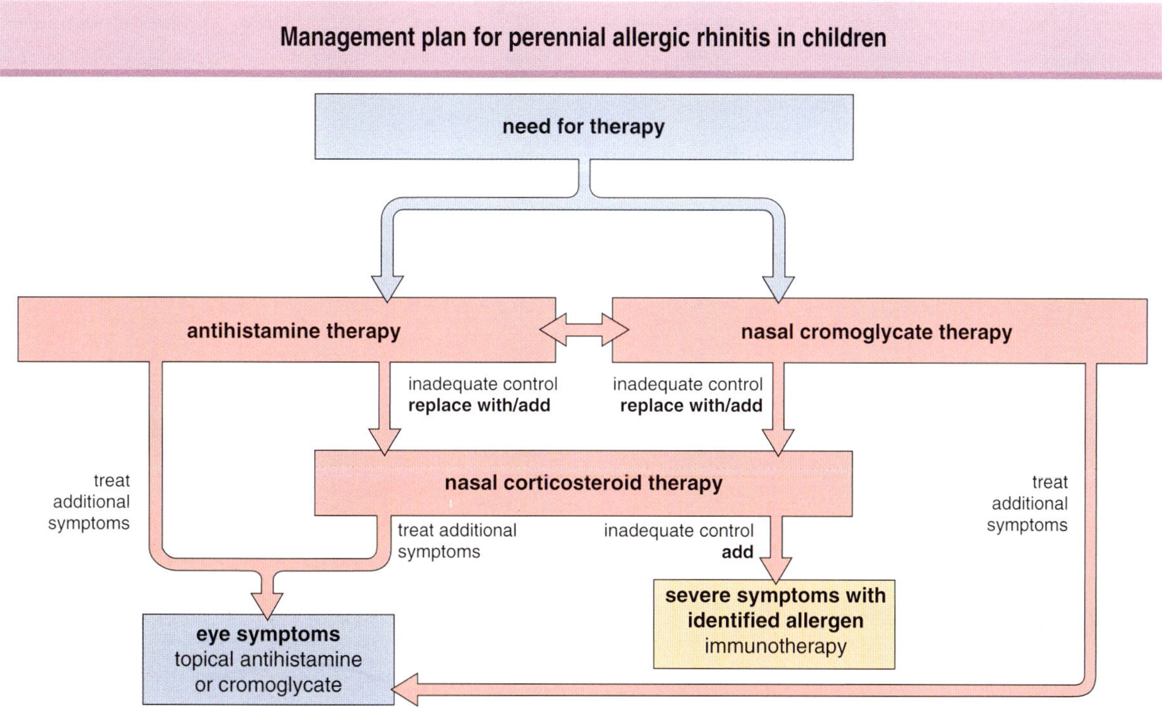

Fig. 1.27 Management plan for perennial allergic rhinitis in children.

Drug profile in the therapy of symptoms of rhinitis

	Sneezing	Rhinorrhoea	Blockage	Reduced sense of smell	Itchy eyes	Itchy throat	Itchy ears
Antihistamines	++(+)	++	(+)	–	+++	++	++
Oral vasoconstrictors	–	–	++	(+)	–	–	–
Nasal vasoconstrictors	–	–	+++	+	–	–	–
Cromoglycate	++	+(+)	+	–	++*	–	–
Intranasal steroids	+++	+++	++(+)	+	(+)	+	+
Systemic steroids	++(+)	++(+)	+++	+++	++	++	++
Ipratropium	–	++	–	–	–	–	–

Fig. 1.28 Drug profile in the therapy of nasal symptoms. *As eyedrops.

antihistamine therapy

Oral preparations

The classical, first-generation H_1 antihistamines all cause some degree of sedation, though they are sometimes used when cost is a decisive factor in the choice of therapy. A low-cost regimen would be a first-generation antihistamine such as chlorpheniramine given at least once daily, with prednisolone tablets added if necessary at the peak of the season.

These drugs have been largely replaced by a second generation of non-sedating (e.g. astemizole, ebastine, loratadine, and terfenadine) or marginally sedating (e.g. acrivastine and cetirizine) antihistamines. Most second-generation antihistamines are rapidly absorbed, and are metabolized by the hepatic cytochrome P-450 system. Cetirizine is metabolized renally. All cross the blood-brain barrier with difficulty as they are less lipophilic than first-generation drugs.

Onset of the antihistamine effect is within 1 hour of oral administration (astemizole is an exception). Non-sedating antihistamines may usually be taken once daily (with the exception of acrivastine, which is given three times daily), so dosing at school or at work is not necessary.

Antihistamines are effective in the treatment of itchy eye and nose, sneezing and watery discharge. They are relatively ineffective in the treatment of nasal blockage. Thus they are more effective in hay fever than in chronic perennial allergic rhinitis, which is characterized by nasal blockage.

Mild disease with occasional symptoms should be treated with oral or topical antihistamines, given as required. This approach may be particularly helpful when eye symptoms predominate. Many patients prefer oral medication, and avoidance of eye drops, which contain preservative, is advisable in contact lens wearers.

When some second-generation antihistamines, e.g. cetirizine, are given in recommended doses, a few susceptible individuals may experience sedation and this may be potentiated by alcohol. Increased appetite and weight gain can occur with some oral preparations (e.g. cyproheptadine, ketotifen, astemizole). Overdosing with terfenadine and astemizole, or their interaction with other drugs, can cause serious ventricular arrhythmias (QT prolongation, *torsades de pointes,* and cardiac arrest). In order to eliminate the risk of life-threatening cardiac arrhythmias, strict guidelines must be followed (**Fig. 1.29**) Ebastine prolongs the QT interval, but not at clinically relevant levels.

Safe use of terfenadine and astemizole
The recommended dose should not be exceeded
Avoid concomitant administration of • ketoconazole and itraconazole • erythromycin and other macrolide antibiotics • other drugs metabolized by cytocrome P-450 3A4
The drugs are contraindicated in patients with significant hepatic dysfunction
Other antihistamines are preferable in patients with cardiac disease
Discuss the potential risks with the patient

Fig. 1.29 Safe use of terfenadine and astemizole. Measures to eliminate the risk of serious cardiac arrhythmias.

Topical preparations

Antihistamines in the form of eye drops are highly effective against itching and have a rapid onset of action. Levocabastine used twice daily is more effective than cromoglycate used four times daily. Concomitant use of eye drops is important in patients treated with nasal steroids.

Levocabastine and azelastine nasal sprays offer quick relief from itching and sneezing and, when used twice daily, can prevent the development of these symptoms. They are probably most useful in mild hay fever and when used before predictable exposure to allergen.

nasal cromoglycate therapy

Sodium cromoglycate (disodium cromoglycate, or cromolyn) has a weak anti-inflammatory activity. It is effective only when used before allergen exposure, and can be used prophylactically as a nasal spray and as eye drops.

Cromoglycate gives a variable degree of symptom amelioration in allergic rhino-conjunctivitis. Because of its relatively short duration of action the drug is administered every four hours, and is therefore associated with poor patient compliance.

Cromoglycate is less effective than topical steroids. The main indication for daily use is perennial allergic rhinitis in children, since the drug is virtually free of recognized side-effects. In these patients it is advisable to try cromoglycate together with an antihistamine.

nasal corticosteroid therapy

Corticosteroids are currently the most potent medications available for the treatment of allergic and non-allergic rhinitis and are being used more frequently. They differ from most other forms of drug therapy in that they suppress the inflammatory process itself, rather than simply treating the effects of the inflammation. These drugs therefore have a significant effect on all symptoms of rhinitis. Intranasal steroids are now considered first-line therapy in moderate to severe cases of hay fever, perennial allergic rhinitis in adults, perennial non-allergic rhinitis, nasal polyposis, and some patients with recurrent sinusitis.

Drugs and drug administration

When a corticosteroid is applied to the nasal mucosa, part of the dose is absorbed into the circulation. However, effective doses are not associated with a significant risk of systemic side-effects.

Beclomethasone dipropionate was introduced in 1974, and flunisolide, budesonide, triamcinolone acetonide, fluticasone propionate, and mometasone furoate followed later. All are effective, though relatively minor differences between the drugs in terms of clinical efficacy have been demonstrated.

Local therapy can be given by metered-dose aqueous pump spray, dry powder inhaler or a CFC-propelled aerosol. (CFC-propelled aerosols are being phased out or replaced by HFA formulations for environmental reasons.) Once-daily medication is usually sufficient and is associated with good patient compliance.

When drugs are administered nasally in children, it is important to teach the correct inhalation technique to ensure an optimal response.

Seasonal allergic rhinitis

Symptom relief in hay fever can be achieved within 6–12 hours, and is maximal after 2–4 days. A steroid spray controls nasal symptoms in the majority of patients but, as with any type of treatment, highly allergic patients can have a symptom breakthrough at the peak of the pollen season. In seasonal allergic rhinitis, regular nasal steroid therapy should ideally be started pre-season to suppress the initiation of the inflammatory response. This may be difficult to arrange in practice, and nasal steroid therapy is very effective in most patients even when started after the onset of symptoms. There is no contraindication to a 2–3 month course of treatment. Thus, nasal steroids can be used as first-line therapy for hay fever in both children and adults.

The choice between a nasal steroid and an antihistamine preparation depends upon the frequency and severity of the symptoms, and whether they are predominantly nasal or conjunctival. Moderate to severe disease with daily nasal symptoms is usually most effectively treated by a nasal steroid plus antihistamine or cromoglycate eye drops.

Perennial rhinitis

Patients with daily symptoms require topical steroid treatment. This is more effective than antihistamines in chronic disease, and particularly where there is nasal blockage.

Patients with perennial allergic rhinitis experience considerable improvement using a nasal steroid, as do most patients with perennial non-allergic rhinitis or nasal polyps.

When nasal blockage is pronounced, a short course of systemic steroid increases the number of responders. However, a subgroup of patients with perennial non-allergic rhinitis seem to be non-responders to any type of steroid treatment. A nasal smear demonstrating eosinophilia usually predicts a good result.

Adverse effects

Nasal irritation and sneezing immediately after spraying are frequent but usually diminish with time. Dryness in the anterior part of the nose, blood-stained crusts and even epistaxis can occur with some preparations, but are not progressive and are seldom troublesome. Dose reduction, use of an ointment in the nostril, and change to an aqueous solution or a powder formulation can be helpful in these cases. Rarely a septal perforation may occur

Safety in children

Although intranasal steroids can be used freely in hay fever, it is the opinion of many paediatricians that regular use of intranasal steroids in children with perennial rhinitis should usually be restricted to cases not controllable by other means (**Fig. 1.30**). Although no clinically significant side-effects on growth or other parameters have been shown to occur when children are treated with nasal steroids in recommended doses, there is a potential risk of mild growth suppression if a child is also receiving inhaled steroid therapy for asthma, as this would increase the total systemic steroid dose. A once-daily dose minimizes the theoretical risk of systemic effects from topical steroid therapy.

Safety during pregnancy

In principle, no medication can be considered 100% safe during pregnancy, especially during the first trimester. The following rules are advisable: (i) prescribe drugs only if absolutely necessary, (ii) prefer topical to systemic administration, and (iii) prefer an old and widely-used drug to a recently launched agent.

Topical nasal steroids have been in use for more than 20 years and have not been associated with any teratogenic or other adverse effects when given in the recommended dosage.

Regular use of nasal steroids in children
Daily symptoms of significance for the child
Allergen avoidance carried out
Cromoglycate and antihistamine insufficient
Medication given once daily in the morning
Keep the daily dose as low as possible
Regular checks

Fig. 1.30 The use of nasal steroids for perennial allergic rhinitis in children.

eye symptoms

Eye itching is a common symptom of hay fever, and approximately one quarter of patients think it more troublesome than the nasal symptoms. Patients who regularly use an oral antihistamine have good protection. Those who use oral antihistamine only when required, and those who are on nasal steroids, will need eye drops to give quick relief from eye itching. Applying eye drops is a good way to avoid eye rubbing and its consequence, a red smarting eye. The antihistamine levocabastine is more effective than cromoglycate, and is fully effective when used twice daily.

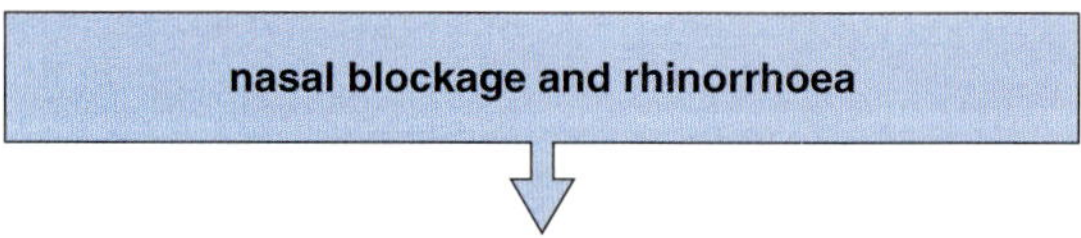

Severe nasal blockage is usually relieved by nasal steroid therapy, but an alpha-adrenergic decongestant given topically or orally can give further relief in selected cases.

Topical decongestants

The potent and long-acting xylometazoline and oxymetazoline, given from metered-dose pump sprays, are easy to use. Patients like the quick onset of action, and the pronounced, prolonged effect (6–8 hours), and may wish to use these drugs long-term. However, long-term treatment results in the development of rhinitis medicamentosa, characterized by rebound congestion and increased nasal irritability. Regular use of intranasal vasoconstrictors must therefore be limited to 7–10 days.

These sprays should only be used in patients with perennial rhinitis and severe nasal blockage, (i) when the patient starts treatment with topical steroid, in order to ensure optimal drug distribution in the nose, and (ii) when the patient has upper airway infection and sinusitis.

Oral decongestants

Oral medication with alpha-adrenoceptor agonists has less effect on nasal patency than topical treatment, but can be used regularly without risk of rhinitis medicamentosa. However, it is not elegant pharmacotherapy to constrict every blood vessel in the body in order to treat a blocked nose, and the dosage needed may cause systemic side-effects (e.g. restlessness, insomnia, tremor, tachycardia, palpitations). There are also many contraindications (e.g. coronary disease, hypertension, prostatism, thyrotoxicosis, glaucoma, diabetes mellitus, and use of monoamine oxidase inbibitors).

Oral preparations of an alpha-agonist plus an antihistamine are widely used for allergic rhinitis. These two drugs complement each other, and their side-effects on the CNS (stimulation and sedation, respectively) tend to be mutually neutralizing.

Ipratropium

Isolated watery rhinorrhoea not associated with sneezing rarely responds to antihistamine or steroid therapy. It is mediated by cholinergic receptors in nasal glands, and can be reduced by topical application of the anticholinergic drug, ipratropium bromide.

This drug is effective in perennial non-allergic rhinitis, but careful selection of patients is necessary as ipratropium is only effective in the treatment of watery rhinorrhoea. It can also inhibit rhinorrhoea induced by cold air ('skier's nose'), hot spicy food ('gustatory rhinitis'), and the common cold.

The dosage of ipratropium must be adjusted to match the severity of symptoms, in order to optimize efficacy and minimize adverse effects such as nasal dryness.

Ipratropium also has an effect on watery rhinorrhoea in allergic rhinitis, but is rarely used as the rhinorrhoea is usually controlled by antihistamines or steroids.

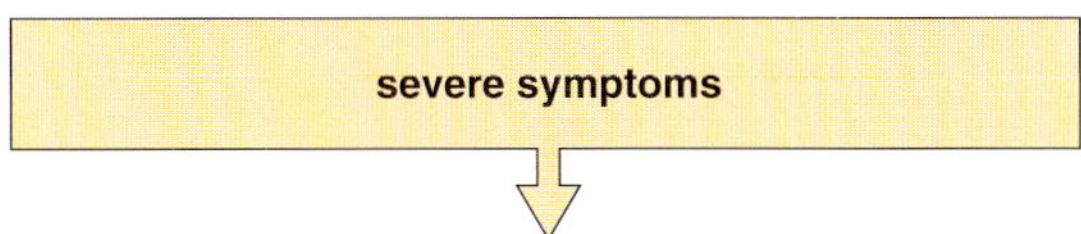

In severe cases of rhinitis, systemic steroids are a valuable supplement to other therapies. A short course can suppress the 'vicious circle' of inflammation and give prolonged relief. When used not more than once every 3–6 months, this treatment is effective and well tolerated.

Preparations

Steroids can be given orally (e.g. prednisolone 5–10 mg/day) or as a depot injection (e.g. methylprednisolone 40–80 mg/injection). Oral treatment should be confined to 2 weeks, which corresponds approximately to the steroid activity of a single depot injection. While many general practitioners use depot injections, most specialists recommend oral medication, as the dose can be adjusted to changing treatment needs, for example during a pollen season with a highly variable pollen count.

Seasonal allergic rhinitis

A short course of systemic steroids (e.g. prednisolone 5–10 mg in the morning) may be given to very sensitive patients when the pollen count is high, and when other treatments are inadequate. This approach may also be valuable to cover specific events, such as school examinations, in patients whose symptoms have not been controlled by other approaches.

Perennial rhinitis and nasal polyposis

Systemic steroids, in contrast to topical treatment, reach all parts of the nose and the paranasal sinuses. Short courses can be used in severe perennial rhinitis or nasal polyposis to open up a blocked nose before or during topical therapy.

Contraindications

Contraindications include glaucoma, herpes keratitis, diabetes mellitus, psychosis, advanced osteoporosis, severe hypertension, and tuberculosis. Systemic steroids are not used for rhinitis in children or during pregnancy.

Side-effects

A 2-week course of treatment is associated with few side-effects, all mild in severity. Depot injections can, in rare cases, cause a depression over the injection site. Some authors recommend depot injections into swollen nasal turbinates and polyps, but this must be discouraged as instances of resulting blindness have been reported.

severe symptoms with identified allergen

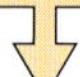

Immunotherapy is an effective treatment for pollen allergy, but opinion varies as to when it should be given, and how often. Most specialists agree that drug treatment should be tried first, and that immunotherapy should be considered only when systemic steroids are needed to control the disease. In perennial allergic rhinitis, immunotherapy can be considered in young, mite-allergic patients with severe rhinitis, and in selected animal-allergic patients. In order to make the treatment as safe as possible, immunotherapy should be limited to specialized centres.

treatment for nasal polyps

The aetiology of nasal polyps is unknown. Although they were formerly considered to be manifestations of an allergic disease, they are not usually associated with any identifiable allergy. The polyps, which consist of an oedematously transformed mucous membrane, are pear-shaped with a stalk originating in the upper part of the nose around the openings to the ethmoidal sinuses (**Fig. 1.31**). Polyposis is typically associated with perennial non-allergic eosinophilic rhinitis, non-allergic asthma and intolerance to acetylsalicylic acid and other NSAIDs. Polyps also occur in patients with cystic fibrosis and primary ciliary dyskinesia.

Therapy for nasal polyposis is a combination of long-term nasal steroid treatment, short-term systemic steroid treatment and, in selected patients, surgical polypectomy. In the small number of patients in whom this combination is unsuccessful, endonasal ethmoidectomy (functional endoscopic sinus surgery or FESS) may be indicated.

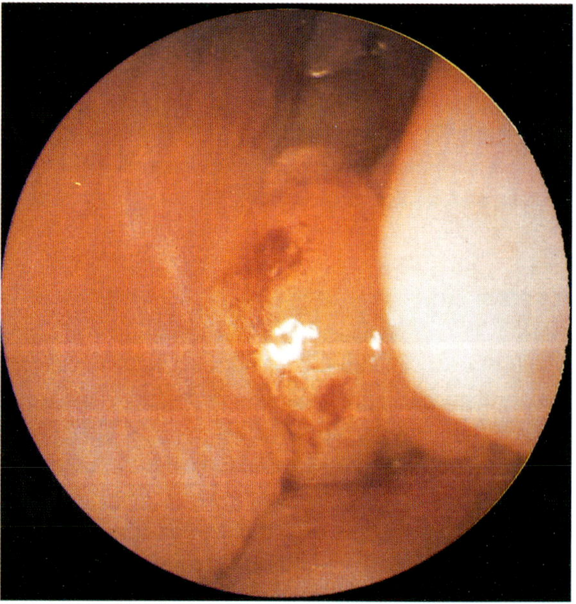

Fig. 1.31 Nasal polyposis seen at endoscopy.

garded as a positive test. This reduction can be reversed with an inhaled bronchodilator.

Airway responsiveness can also be measured as the reaction to non-specific inhaled agents such as histamine and methacholine (**Fig. 2.8**). Although there is considerable overlap between groups, there is a trend to increased bronchial responsiveness moving from normal individuals through patients with hay fever to mild, moderate, and severe asthma. Avoidance of allergens, or use of anti-inflammatory asthma drugs, can reduce this responsiveness. Measurement of airway responsiveness can be useful in difficult cases but is not necessary in the routine assessment of asthma.

Chest X-ray examination may be useful to exclude other

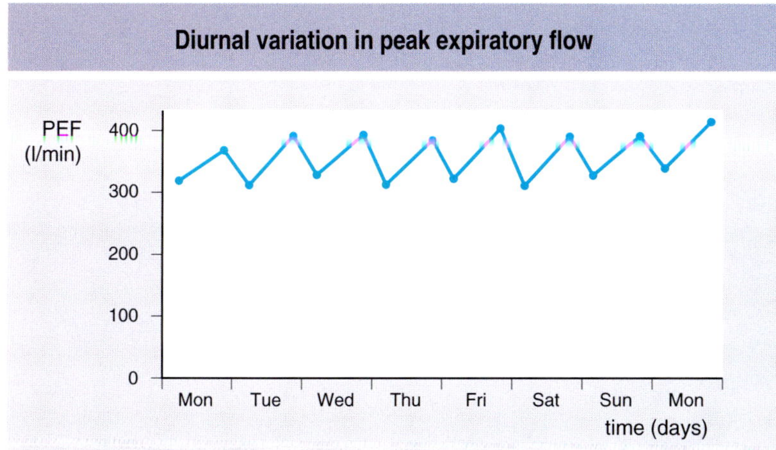

Fig. 2.6 Diurnal variation in peak expiratory flow. A small variation between morning (lower) and evening (higher) values is commonly seen in normal subjects but diurnal variability above 15% is diagnostic of asthma.

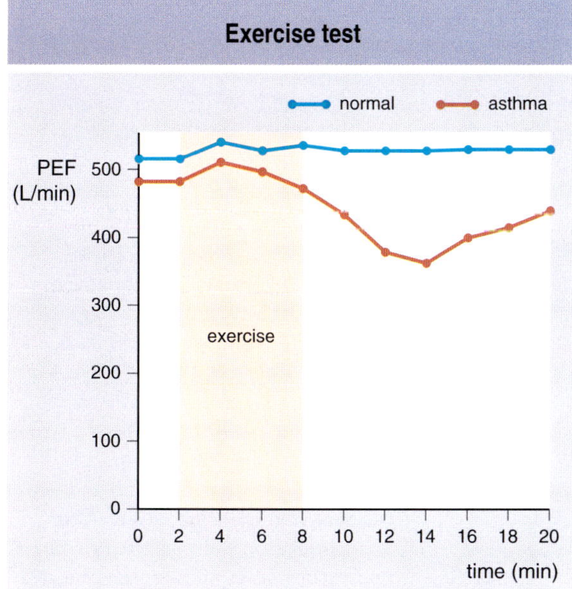

Fig. 2.7 Exercise test. Peak flow often rises a little during exercise but may begin to fall before the end of the standard 6-minute exercise period. A positive test has a drop in PEF of at least 15%.

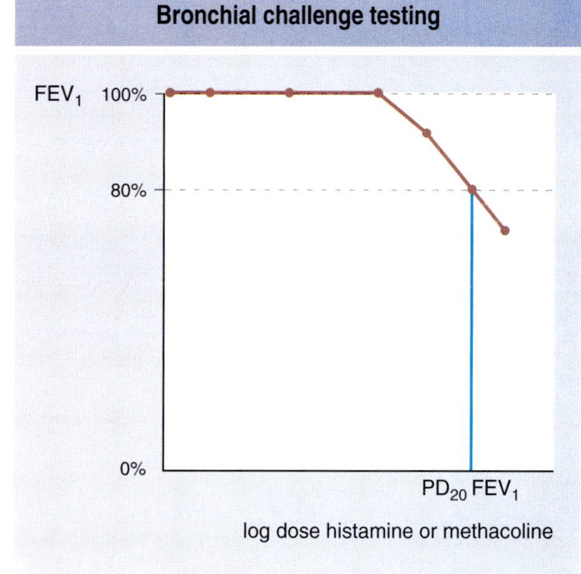

Fig. 2.8 Airway responsiveness. Challenge tests with allergen may also provoke late reactions but these are not seen with histamine or methacholine.

diagnoses but is not helpful in the diagnosis of asthma itself. Skin prick tests and radioallergosorbent tests detect specific IgE and may help to confirm trigger factors for asthma (*see* **Fig. 1.22 & 1.23**). A positive response to either of these tests confirms the atopic predisposition to develop asthma.

Spirometry provides an alternative to peak flow measurement, giving a measure of forced expiratory volume in one second (FEV_1) and forced vital capacity (FVC) (**Fig 2.9**). A low forced expiratory ratio (FEV_1/FVC) indicates airflow obstruction. The same information can be supplied as a plot of flow against volume in the flow–volume curve. Early airflow obstruction appears as reduced flow at lower lung volumes before there is much of an effect on peak flow (**Fig. 2.10**).

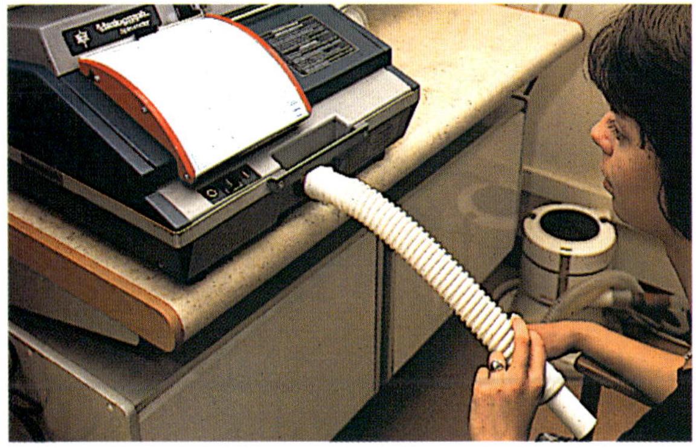

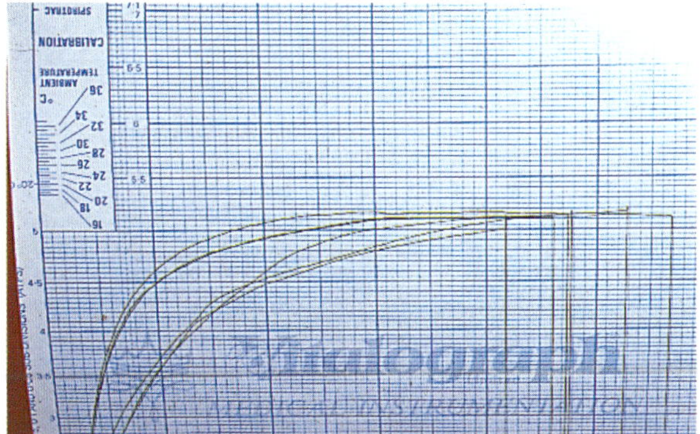

Fig. 2.9 Spirometry. In the forced expired vital capacity manoeuvre, the patient takes a maximal inspiration and is then asked to exhale as fast as possible for as long as possible. The volume expired against time is measured and the forced expired volume in one second (FEV_1) can be determined, as can the forced vital capacity (FVC). The ratio of FEV_1/FVC if reduced (less than 75%, suggests airflow obstruction, but each variate can be assessed against predicted values, which depend on sex, age, height and ethnic origin (see also Fig. 2.5). Respiratory function laboratories usually measure FEV_1/FVC using bellows-type spirometers, but increasingly smaller turbine or other electronic devices are used.

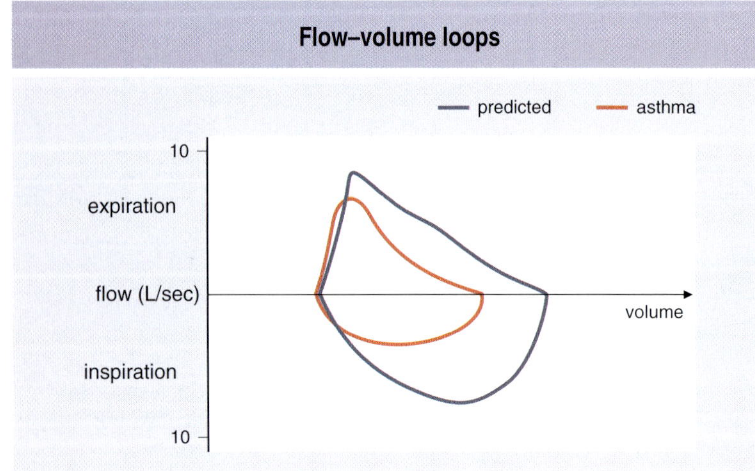

Fig. 2.10 Flow–volume loops. The forced expiratory manoeuvre can also be displayed as flow against volume. Conventionally volume is displayed on the horizontal axis. A maximum inspiratory breath can be included to give the full loop. In asthma both inspiratory flow and expiratory flow are reduced and the residual volume is increased. After a bronchodilator the expiratory and inspiratory flows should increase and residual volume and total lung capacity may decrease. Changes in lung volume may produce symptomatic improvement with minimal increases in FEV_1 or FVC.

Exclude other causes of wheezing

The main differential diagnosis is chronic obstructive pulmonary disease (COPD). Around 20% of smokers suffer an accelerated decline in lung function which ends in symptomatic COPD (chronic bronchitis and/or emphysema) if they continue to smoke. The majority of smokers are not susceptible to COPD although they retain the risks of cardiovascular disease, as well as lung and other cancers, from their smoking. Cough and sputum are symptoms that occur more often in smokers than the obstructive problems of COPD.

COPD may be difficult to differentiate from chronic asthma in adults. Occasionally asthma may go unrecognized by patient and doctor and even present with right heart failure secondary to chronic hypoxia and pulmonary hypertension. A history of smoking is usual in COPD and the degree of reversibility with bronchodilators and steroids is less than in asthma.

The main purpose of differentiation from COPD is to ensure appropriate treatment. Asthmatics with persistent symptoms should receive anti-inflammatory treatment while the role of regular steroids in COPD remains uncertain.

Large airway obstruction may occasionally be misdiagnosed as asthma. The clue to correct diagnosis comes from the detection of a monophonic wheeze. The diagnosis can be confirmed by the flow–volume curve, which shows a low flow throughout expiration and inspiration (**Fig. 2.11**).

Monitor the condition

The provision of a portable peak flow meter will allow a patient to monitor his or her asthma. This should form part of a management plan that gives guidance on when to adjust therapy, and when to seek medical assistance. Used in this way, portable peak flow meters can improve control of the disease. Management plans should be developed in partnership with the patient, and should take into account their personal circumstances, level of education, and so on. Special emphasis should be placed on the importance of correct inhaler technique and compliance, as studies have shown that approximately 50% of prescribed asthma drugs are not used as directed. The aims of asthma treatment are summarized in **Fig. 2.12**.

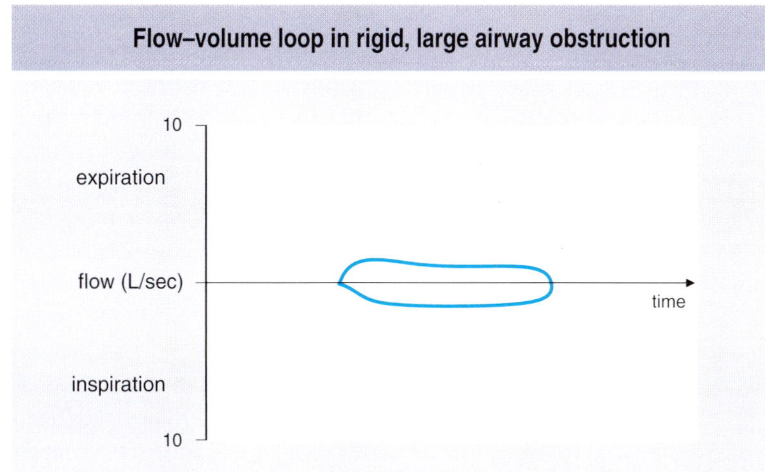

Fig. 2.11 Flow–volume loop in rigid, large airway obstruction. The characteristic fixed low flow in expiration and inspiration results from rigid narrowing by malignancy in the trachea or external pressure on the trachea from a mass such as a retrosternal goitre.

Aims of treatment in chronic asthma
To prevent or minimize symptoms, rather than to treat them as they occur
To permit normal activities in daily life
To achieve normal or best-possible lung function
To limit β_2-agonist therapy to occasional rather than regular use
To avoid side-effects from therapy
To prevent exacerbations

Fig. 2.12 Aims of treatment in chronic asthma.

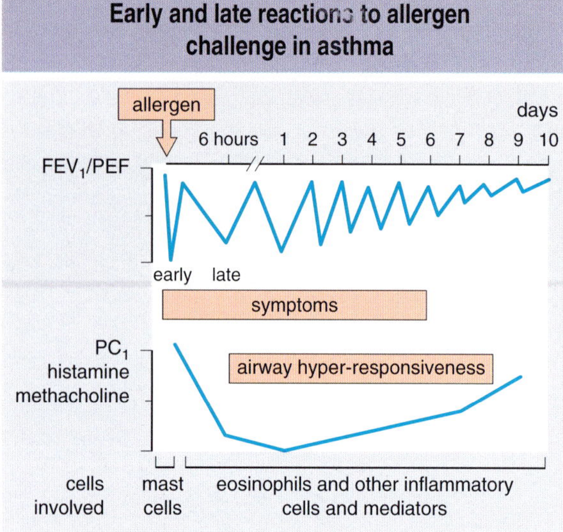

Fig. 2.13 Early and late reactions to allergen challenge in asthma. In the laboratory, patients can be exposed to a single large dose of allergen. This results in an immediate, short-lived decline in lung function as measured by the forced expiratory volume in 1 second (FEV_1) or the peak expiratory flow (PEF). The decline is commonly followed within 6 hours or more by a late-phase reaction. The early reaction is usually reversible by inhaled bronchodilator therapy, but the late reaction is much less readily reversed. Symptoms of asthma may persist for several days, especially at night, and PEF readings may show low early morning values ('morning dipping'). Over the same period, there is an increase in airway responsiveness, as measured by histamine or methacholine challenge tests. Mast cells have a predominant role in the immediate reaction to allergen challenge, but other inflammatory cells and mediators have the predominant role in the prolonged late reaction.

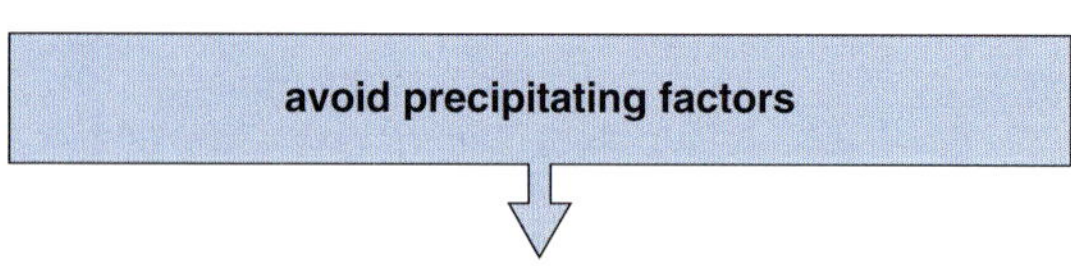

In most cases asthma needs drug treatment. However, every attempt should be made to avoid known precipitating factors ('triggers'). Most asthmatics have multiple sensitivities so that total avoidance is not possible. Even so, avoiding major triggers is likely to improve control or limit the extent of drug therapy required. Exposure to an allergen can worsen control and increase general responsiveness to other triggers for several days afterwards (**Fig. 2.13**).

Some patients have single specific precipitants for asthma, so that identification and exclusion of the allergen effectively 'cures' the asthma. There is a significant occupational element in at least 5% of all cases (**Fig. 2.14**). This should be sought by detailed history, with peak flow records taken both at work and away from work. Drugs (**Fig. 2.15**), such as β-blockers, aspirin and non-steroidal anti-inflammatory agents, are common precipitants. Allergens from pets are also common triggers, and can often be relatively easily avoided or removed (**Fig. 2.16**).

Non-specific inhaled triggers can worsen asthma control. Active and passive smoking must be avoided. Various other pollutants (e.g. industrial by-products, traffic fumes) can worsen asthma. This might influence the choice of housing or occupation.

Some agents provoking occupational asthma	
Isocyanates	Tea dust
Soldering flux (colophony)	Wood dust
Stainless steel welding	Laboratory animals and insects
Platinum salts	Animals/insects, larval forms
Epoxy resin hardening agents	Crustaceans
Azodicarbonamide (PVC, plastics)	Flour/grain dust
Glutaraldehyde (sterilization procedures in hospitals)	Castor bean dust
Persulphate salts	Soya bean dust
Reactive dyes	Green coffee beans
Proteolytic enzymes (washing powder manufacture)	Drug manufacture (antibiotics, cimetidine, ipecacuanha, ispaghula)

Fig. 2.14 Some agents provoking occupational asthma. The list of agents officially recognized for industrial injury compensation varies between countries.

Drugs which may provoke asthma
All beta-blockers (including eye drops)
Aspirin and NSAIDs
Penicillins
Inhaled drugs
ACE inhibitors
Adenosine
Iodine-containing contrast media

Fig. 2.15 Drugs which may provoke asthma.

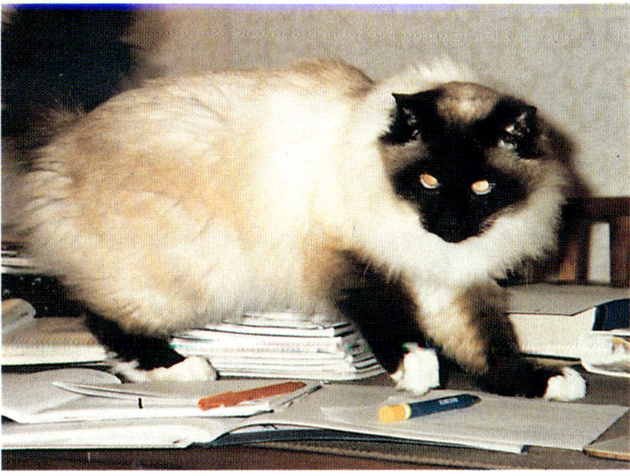

Fig. 2.16 Allergy to cats is common in patients with asthma. Cats and other animals should always be banished from bedrooms and ideally from the patient's home.

inhaled bronchodilators as needed

Bronchodilators should be used as needed for symptoms such as wheeze, shortness of breath and cough. They should also be used 15–30 minutes before exercise where this is known to provoke asthma.

Inhaled short-acting β_2-receptor agonists are the relief bronchodilator class of choice in mild intermittent asthma, where symptoms occur less than once a day. A number of drugs are available, with minor differences in speed of onset and length of action. Salbutamol and terbutaline are the most commonly used agents in many countries.

There is some evidence to suggest that the regular use of β_2-agonists may cause a minor increase in airway responsiveness, and thus worsen control. Published guidelines therefore do not recommend the use of bronchodilators for regular treatment without the concurrent use of anti-inflammatory agents, and β_2-agonists alone are no longer considered appropriate therapy for patients with chronic asthma and regular symptoms. If patients have more than occasional mild symptoms, or use β_2-agonists on most days, then they should also have regular treatment with an inhaled steroid.

The most common adverse effects of inhaled β_2-agonists such as salbutamol and terbutaline are tremor, tachycardia and muscle cramps. In most cases these are minor inconveniences and decline with regular use of the drug. For the occasional patient with persistent problems, an anticholinergic bronchodilator such as ipratropium bromide can be used. Anticholinergic agents have a slower onset and are generally less effective than β_2-agonists in asthma.

There is a wide choice of inhalation devices. These fall in to two main groups: pressurized metered dose inhalers (pMDIs) and dry-powder inhalers (DPIs). Traditional pMDIs **(Fig. 2.17)** use chlorofluorocarbons (CFCs) as propellants and contribute to depletion of the stratospheric ozone layer. A new generation of pMDIs containing hydrofluoroalkane (HFA) propellants are now becoming available.. These alternative propellants which are not damaging to the ozone layer will replace CFCs over the next few years. Most adult patients are able to use pMDIs efficiently after adequate training. Those who cannot co-ordinate activation of the inhaler with inspiration can use a spacing device with the pMDI **(Fig. 2.18)**, a breath actuated inhaler **(Fig. 2.19)** or a DPI. DPIs come in various forms, the most convenient

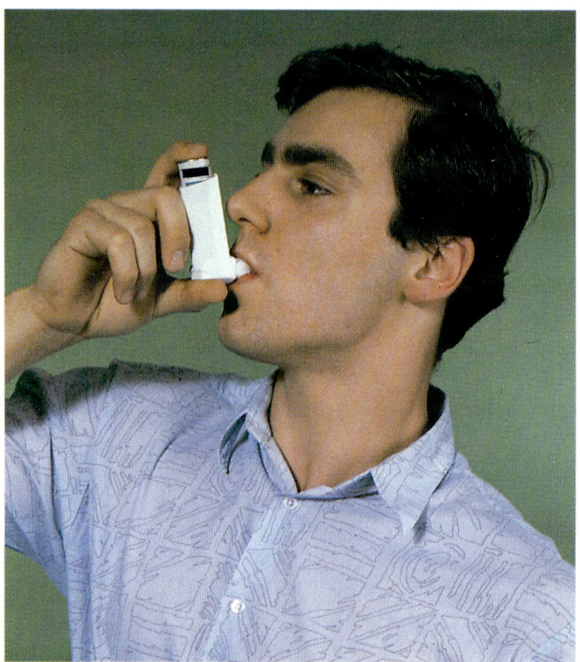

Fig. 2.17 A pressurized metered dose inhaler (pMDI). A metered dose of drug is released on pressing down the canister against a spring-loaded valve. Many patients have difficulty in co-ordinating actuation of the inhaler with inspiration, so training and monitoring in the successful use of such inhalers is essential. Conventional pMDIs, which contain CFC propellants, are being phased out for environmental reasons.

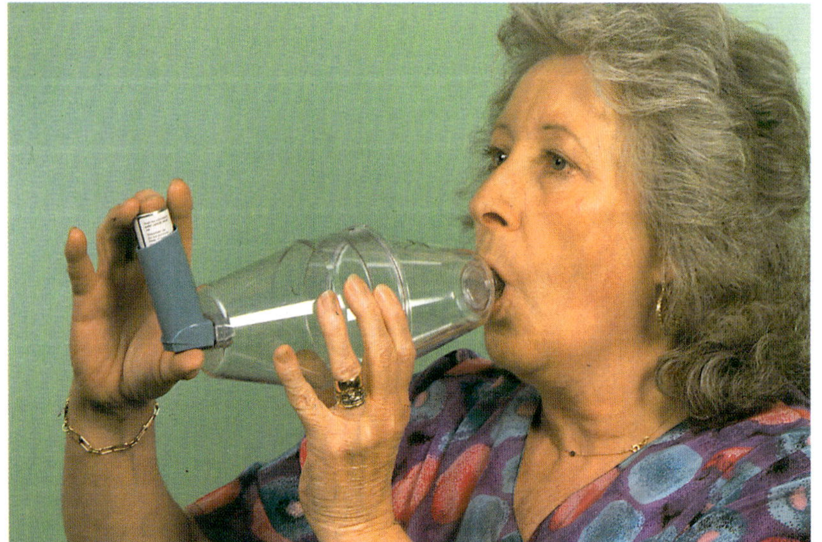

Fig. 2.18 Large volume 'spacer' or extension chamber added to a pMDI. Large volume spacers have a one-way respiratory valve, which helps to overcome co-ordination problems, especially in children. Such spacer devices may also increase lung deposition and reduce oropharyngeal impaction of drug aerosol – features which are particularly useful when high-dose inhaled steroid therapy is used.

contain multiple doses and are simple to use **(Figs 2.20 & 2.21)**. The same range of inhalation devices is available for β2-agonists and steroids. Inhalation technique should be checked regularly as part of the management of all asthmatics.

Note that different devices deliver a different proportion of the nominal dose to the lungs, so prescriptions should specify the drug, the dose and the delivery device or system to be used.

regular anti-inflammatory agent (usually inhaled steroid)

The step up from occasional bronchodilator use is the addition of a regular inhaled anti-inflammatory drug with continuation of the inhaled bronchodilator as needed. Inhaled steroids are the most widely used and effective anti-inflammatory agents in this step.

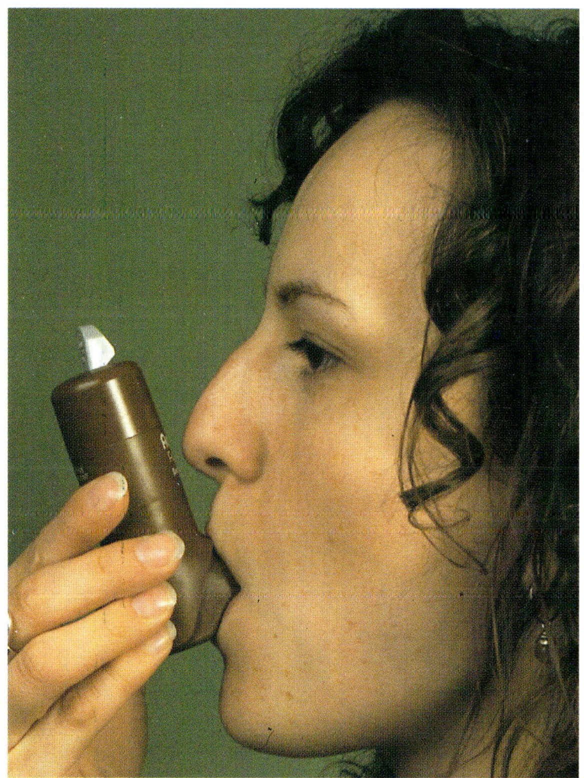

Fig. 2.19 Breath-actuated pMDI. Breath-actuated devices are triggered by the start of inspiration by the patient. They help to overcome the problem of poor co-ordination, and are actuated by such low inspiratory flow rates that they can be used to deliver rescue therapy in acute severe asthma.

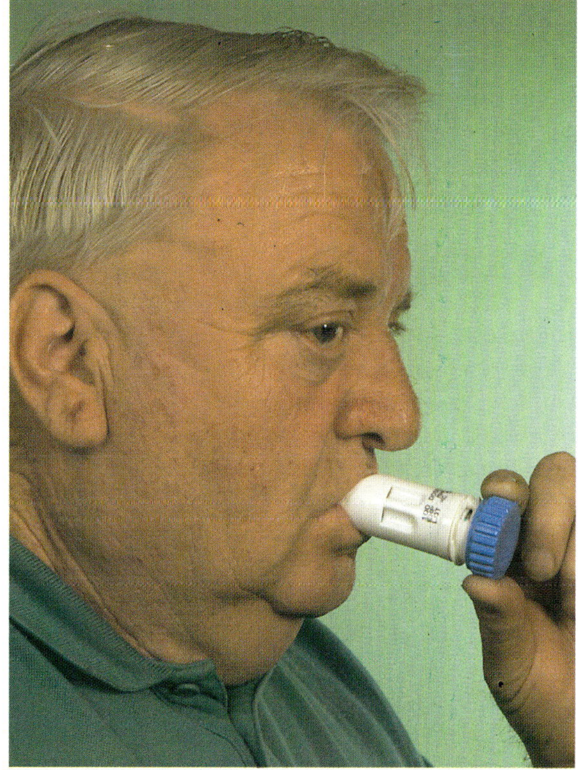

Fig. 2.20 A dry-powder, multidose inhaler (Turbohaler or Turbuhaler). Dry-powder inhalers are inspiratory flow-actuated and driven, so they overcome the co-ordination problems of pMDIs. The performance of different dry-powder inhalers varies, but Turbohaler achieves a substantially higher lung deposition of drug than pMDI. A single inhaler holds up to 200 doses of the drug.

regular anti-inflammatory agent (usually inhaled steroid)

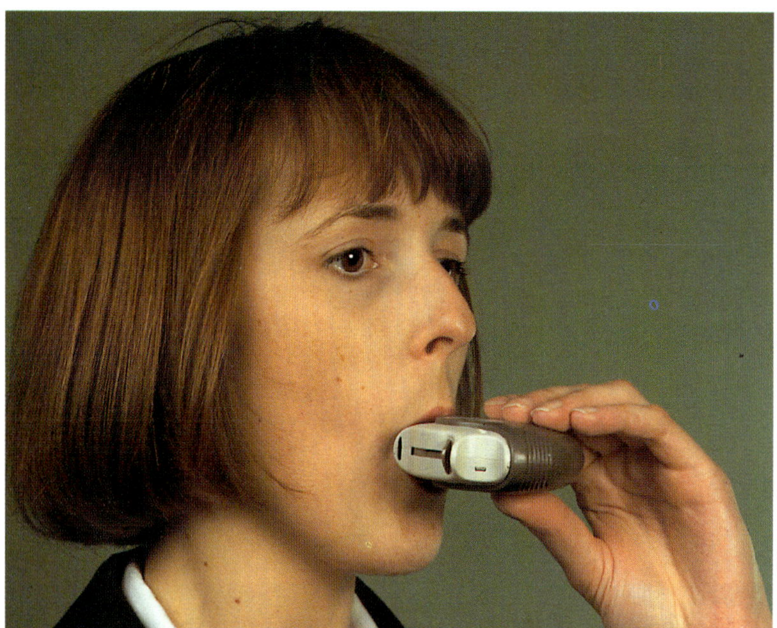

Fig. 2.21 A dry-powder, multidose inhaler (Accuhaler or Diskus). In this inhaler, doses of drug are sealed between two strips of material at regular intervals, so a roll of doses is fitted inside. On actuation, the two strips of material are separated, releasing free drug to the mouth piece where it can be inhaled. A dose counter shows the number of doses remaining in the inhaler.

Alternative agents are sodium cromoglycate and nedocromil sodium. Sodium cromoglycate is used more often in children, where the anxiety over potential adverse effects of inhaled steroids is greater. In both adults and children these alternative agents have less of an effect than inhaled steroids. They may be useful in mild cases, and in patients who are reluctant to use inhaled steroids despite assurances regarding their low potential for systemic effects. Treatment for 2–3 months is necessary to assess the effectiveness of sodium cromoglycate and nedocromil sodium.

Inhaled steroids are used twice daily in most cases. At low doses it is possible to maintain control with once-daily administration. In patients in whom higher doses are required, it may be helpful to split the dose into two, three or four administrations.

Inhaled steroids used in this way provide good control in most cases of mild to moderate asthma, alleviating symptoms and minimizing the need for bronchodilators. There is some evidence to suggest that the early use of inhaled steroids may have a beneficial effect on the natural history of asthma. The suppression of inflammation in the airways, which has been shown

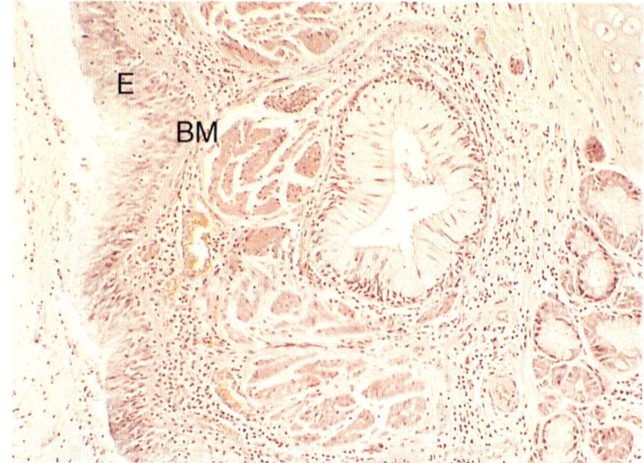

Fig. 2.22 Large airway wall from a fatal case of asthma. The lumen is to the left, and contains a mucus plug. The epithelium (E) is disrupted, the basement membrane (BM) is thickened, there is widespread infiltration with inflammatory cells, smooth muscle hyperplasia and hypertrophy of the mucus glands (to the right). Inhaled steroid therapy has been shown to reverse the inflammatory changes in asthma, and early use of inhaled steroids may prevent the structural changes shown here. Original magnification ×25.

wheezing in association with upper respiratory tract infections once or twice a year.

A substantial minority of patients, perhaps 20%, have a poor perception of changes in their own airway calibre. In such patients symptoms may be an unreliable guide to their condition and they may be at particular risk of severe life-threatening exacerbations. Extra attention needs to be paid to objective monitoring with peak flow meters when these 'poor perceivers' are identified.

Cough may be the only presenting feature of asthma. This is most common in children when sleep disturbance by coughing is common and may be misdiagnosed and mistreated as an infective problem.

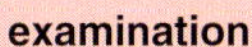

examination

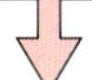

The main finding on examination in asthma is wheeze on auscultation. Wheezes are best heard on expiration when there is relative narrowing of the intrathoracic airways, but they are often also audible on inspiration. Wheezes are heard at various pitches reflecting the widespread airway narrowing. A single monophonic wheeze raises the suspicion of a large airway narrowing. In periods of remission there are likely to be no abnormal findings on routine examination.

Acute exacerbations of asthma are associated with overinflation of the thorax. In chronic severe asthma this overinflation may be persistent.

There may be evidence on examination of associated atopic conditions such as flexural eczema or rhinitis. Nasal polyps may be associated with asthma, particularly later onset asthma with aspirin sensitivity.

A simple estimation of airway calibre such as peak expiratory flow should be regarded as a normal part of the clinical examination of the patient.

make the diagnosis

The diagnosis of asthma may be evident from the history. Confirmation relies on a demonstration of the variability of airflow obstruction. This is done most easily with a traditional Wright peak flow meter (**Fig. 2.2**), or one of the cheaper portable versions (**Fig. 2.3**). The value recorded is the highest of three technically satisfactory measurements made as a maximal expiration from total

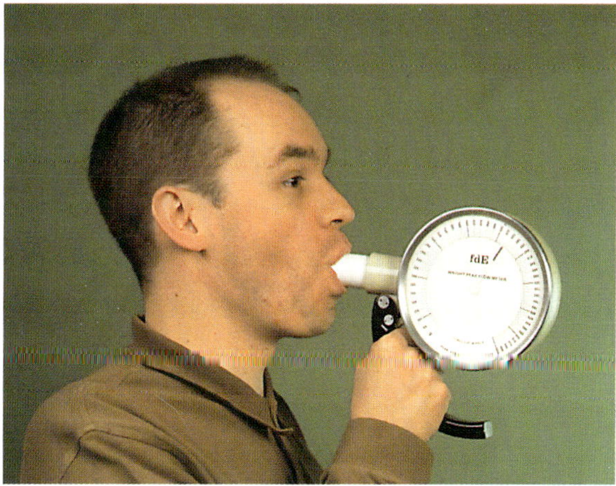

Fig. 2.2 Wright's peak flow meter. This is the standard peak expiratory flow meter used in most respiratory function laboratories. After a maximal inspiration the patient is asked to make a short sharp expiration as fast as possible. The meter registers the maximal flow sustained for 10 milliseconds. Few patients are unable to carry out this test. The procedure is repeated to obtain three technically satisfactory blows and the maximum value taken.

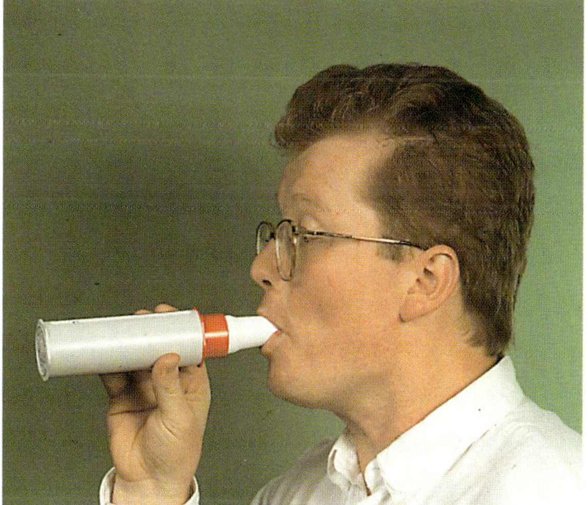

Fig. 2.3 Portable 'mini-Wright' peak flow meter. A number of inexpensive, portable devices are available for the measurement of peak flow at home.

2 Chronic Asthma

P John Rees

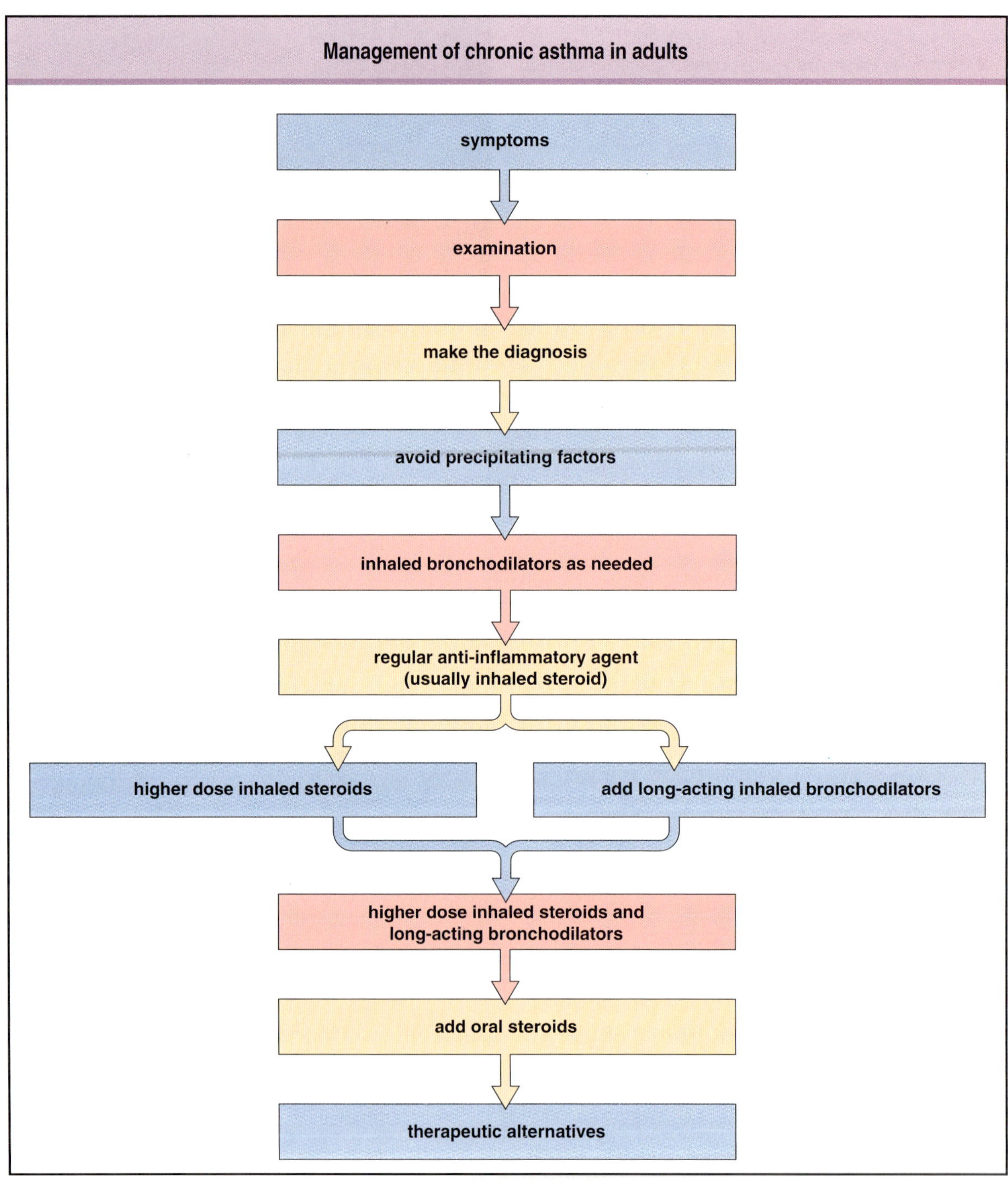

lung capacity. Predicted values are shown in **Fig. 2.4**.

The administration of an inhaled bronchodilator (e.g. a fast-acting, selective β_2-agonist) can be used as a diagnostic test for asthma. The response is measured after 15 minutes. Significant bronchodilation is indicated by an increase of 70 L/min in peak flow, or an increase of 200 ml in FEV_1 (**Fig. 2.5**).

If the peak flow is normal, or if there is no significant acute bronchodilator response, then recordings can be made over a longer period. Home recordings are taken at set times, two to four times daily. Diurnal variation is calculated as the mean daily difference between morning and evening values (**Fig. 2.6**). Whereas a small variation occurs in normal subjects, diurnal variability above 15% is diagnostic of asthma.

An alternative approach is to look at the ease of inducibility of obstruction. The simplest test is the response to exercise, which causes drying and cooling of the airway mucosa. Vigorous exercise is performed for 6 minutes. In the laboratory this is usually done on a braked static bicycle or a treadmill but the test can be performed quite easily with free running. The exercise response will be increased if it is performed in cold, dry conditions. Peak flow is measured at intervals of 1 or 2 minutes, before, during and after exercise (**Fig. 2.7**). The readings may go up during the exercise period.

A reduction of 15% from baseline after exercise is re-

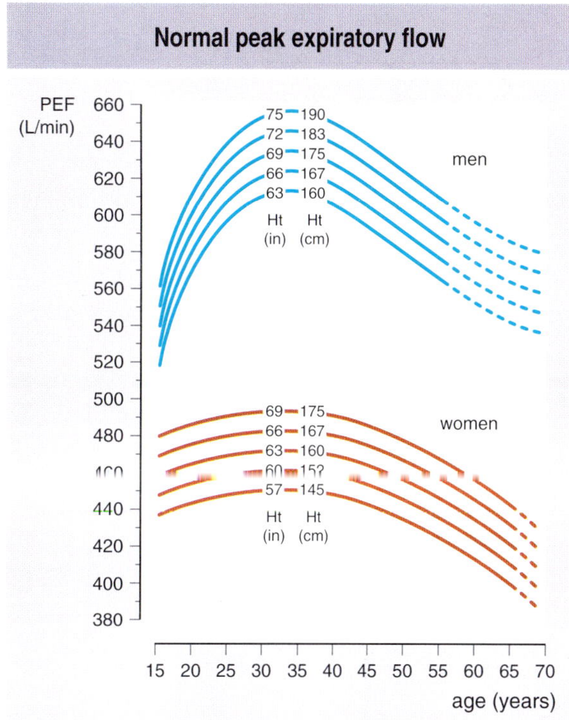

Fig. 2.4 Normal peak expiratory flow. The chart shows the normal values for peak flow rate in men and women between 15 and 70 years. The confidence intervals around the normal values are 100 L/min in men and 85 L/min in women.

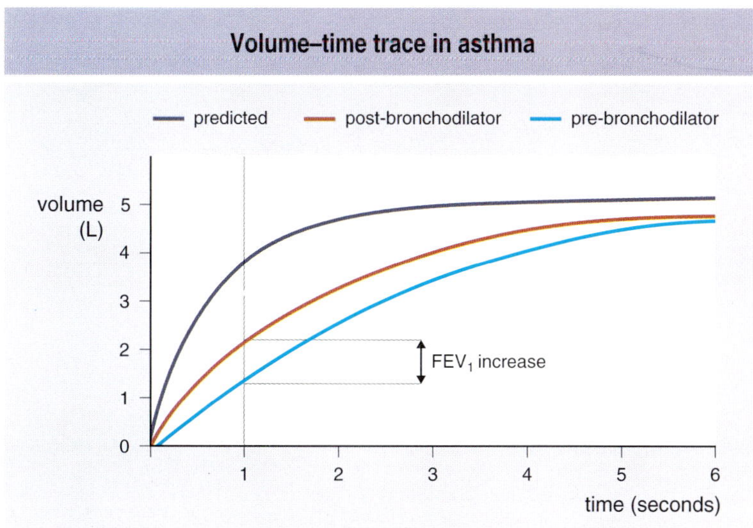

Fig. 2.5 Volume–time trace in asthma, produced by asking the patient to perform forced expiration through a spirometer. In a normal subject ('predicted' value for the age, sex and height of the patient), the vital capacity is expelled in less than 5 seconds, and around 75% of the vital capacity is expelled after 1 second (FEV_1). In asthma, the FEV_1 is reduced to a greater extent than any reduction in the forced vital capacity (FVC). Significant bronchodilation after the administration of an inhaled β_2-agonist is indicated by an increase of at least 200 ml in FEV_1.

2 Chronic Asthma

P John Rees

Asthma is a condition that can cause problems at any time of life. Throughout the world there is evidence of an increase in the prevalence of asthma, exceeding 20% in some studies of children. In some countries the mortality rate is continuing to rise, although it has plateaued or even fallen slightly in others. Recent research has emphasized the importance of inflammation in the wall of the airways as a fundamental component of asthma. The approach to therapy concentrates on the suppression of this inflammation.

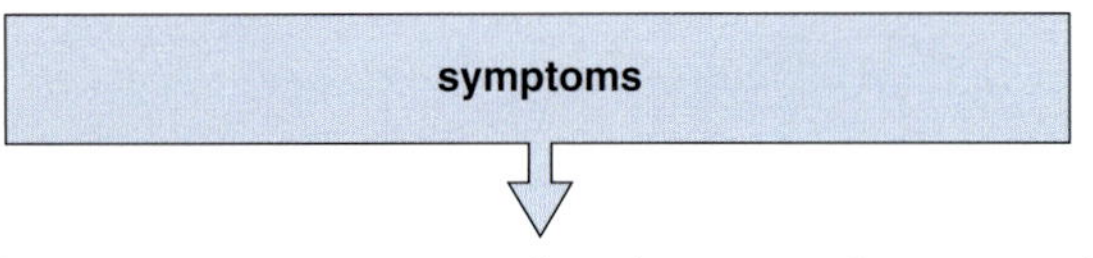

The common symptoms of asthma are shortness of breath, audible wheeze, and cough. A major feature of asthma is the variability of symptoms, either with treatment or spontaneously with time. Increases in breathlessness may occur in response to identifiable triggers (**Fig. 2.1**).

Nocturnal symptoms are a characteristic feature related to the diurnal variability of airway calibre found in many asthmatic patients. In long-standing, poorly controlled asthma this variability may be lost as the airway narrowing and symptoms become persistent.

Breathlessness may be more marked on inspiration or expiration. This is because the airways in the lungs are narrower during expiration, while higher lung volumes mean that more inspiratory work is necessary to breathe in a given volume on inspiration.

The range of severity of asthma is very great, from patients who are always restricted in the performance of minor daily activities to those who develop minimal

Common triggers in asthma		
Allergens:	house dust mite	Exercise
	pollens	
	fungi	Climate
	pets	
	food and drink	Pollution
Drugs		Smoking
Occupational exposure		Emotion
Infections		Gastro-oesophageal reflux

Fig. 2.1 Common triggers in asthma

in biopsies (**Fig. 2.22**) and airway secretions, may reduce the likelihood of the development of irreversible structural changes in the airways. This possibility is under investigation. Meanwhile the widespread use of steroids is justified by their effect on control of asthma symptoms and reduction in exacerbations.

Beclomethasone dipropionate or budesonide are the most common starting drugs and are essentially equivalent when administered by pMDI at lower doses. The usual starting dose is 400–800 μg daily. It is best to start at the higher end of the dose range to establish control, and then reduce the dose for maintenance. Increasing the dose for 1–2 weeks in the event of an upper respiratory tract infection may be useful, although there is no strong evidence for the effectiveness of this approach.

In adults the only clinically significant adverse effects of steroids in doses up to 800 μg daily are local pharyngeal effects. The incidence of oropharyngeal candidiasis (**Fig. 2.23**) can be reduced by use of a large volume spacer with a pMDI, or by rinsing the mouth and spitting out after use of DPIs.

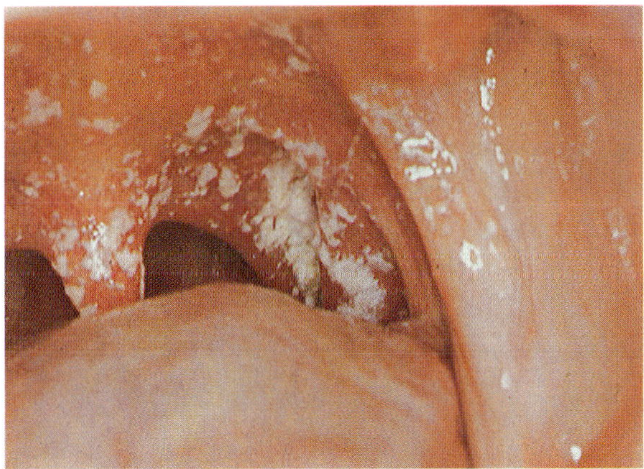

Fig. 2.23 Oropharyngeal candidiasis in a patient receiving inhaled steroid therapy. This complication probably results from the impaction of aerosol particles in the oropharynx, leading to a topical steroid effect and increased local susceptibility to candida infection. The incidence of oropharyngeal candidiasis can be reduced by the use of a large volume spacer with a pMDI, or by rinsing the mouth and spitting out after the use of DPIs. Both these manoeuvres lessen the amount of oropharyngeal deposition of aerosol.

Inhaled bronchodilators should be continued as needed together with regular inhaled steroids. It is important to ensure that patients recognize the different aims of the regular anti-inflammatory inhaler and the relief bronchodilator.

higher dose inhaled steroids

If lower doses of inhaled steroid (400–800 μg/day) fail to establish control of asthma then there are two main strategies. The traditional approach has been to increase the dose of the inhaled steroid up to 1000–2000 μg daily. The alternative approach is to add a long-acting bronchodilator to the lower dose of inhaled steroid.

When the daily dose of inhaled steroid exceeds 1000μg daily then the possibility of adverse effects needs to be considered. Purpura and skin fragility may occur with higher doses of inhaled steroids. Biochemical evidence of effects on the hypophyseal–pituitary–adrenal axis can be found and it may be advisable to give a boost of oral steroids before an operation or with other severe stress, although there are very few reports of clinically significant adrenal suppression with inhaled steroids. Other long-term adverse effects, such as osteoporosis and cataracts, have been suggested but not confirmed. The assessment of these risks is complicated by the fact that most patients with severe asthma also receive courses of oral steroid therapy at some stage in their treatment. At doses of 1000 μg or more, a large volume spacer should be used with pMDIs, and mouth rinsing should be performed following dosing with DPIs; these techniques minimize the amount of steroid deposited in the oropharynx and swallowed.

At higher doses of inhaled steroids it may be advisable to use budesonide or fluticasone, both of which have been shown to undergo substantial 'first pass metabolism' (**Fig. 2.24**). If these drugs are deposited in the mouth and swallowed they are largely metabolized in the liver, so systemic effects from this route are unlikely. However, drug deposited in the respiratory tract enters the systemic circulation without passing through the liver. With currently available inhaled steroids, a potential for systemic effects – however small – is inseparable from their desired clinical effects.

Bronchodilator drugs should be continued as required with higher dose inhaled steroids. The need for

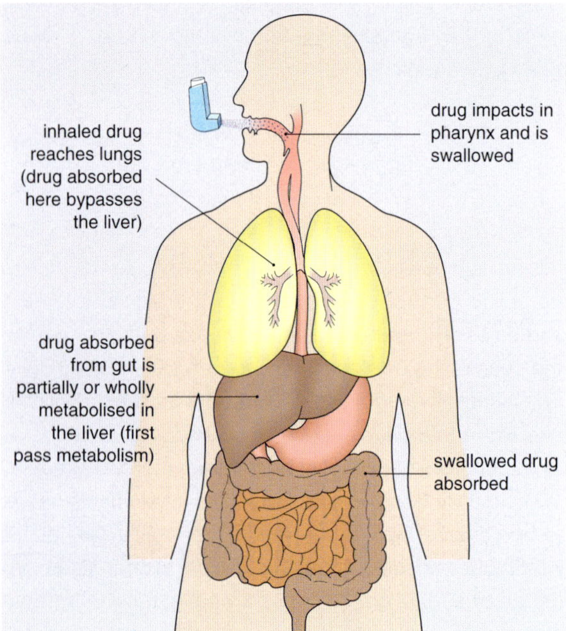

Fig. 2.24 The systemic availability of an inhaled drug is the sum of its absorption from the gastrointestinal and respiratory tracts. After absorption via the gut wall and liver, intact drug which escapes first-pass metabolism reaches the systemic circulation. Absorption via the lungs results in the direct entry of the drug into the systemic circulation. For inhaled steroids with very high first-pass metabolism (e.g. fluticasone, budesonide), this means that most systemic activity results from the portion of the dose deposited in the lungs.

bronchodilators can be used as an indicator of the adequacy of asthma control.

add long-acting inhaled bronchodilators

Oral long-acting bronchodilators have been available for some years but their use has been limited by their adverse effects. Oral β_2-agonists are associated with a high incidence of tremor. Oral theophyllines are effective bronchodilators and have been used for many years. The sustained-release preparations of theophylline allow stable serum concentrations to be achieved but it is necessary to monitor these concentrations and to be aware of possible interactions with other drugs (**Fig. 2.25**). The incidence of adverse effects, particularly nausea and vomiting, is high. It has been suggested that theophyllines at lower doses may have a beneficial antiinflammatory effect, but this has not yet been demonstrated in clinical studies.

The appropriate long-acting bronchodilators at this stage of management are inhaled salmeterol and formoterol. They are effective for more than 12 hours, making them particularly useful for nocturnal symptoms. Prolonged studies show that any long-term loss of bronchodilator effect (tachyphylaxis) is minimal and not clinically significant. However, there does appear to be a reduction in the protective effect against triggered bronchoconstriction with regular use. Initial anxieties that this might leave patients at risk of sudden severe asthma

Factors affecting metabolism of theophyline

Increased clearance	Decreased clearance	
Cigarette smoking	Enzyme inhibition:	erythromycin
		cimetidine
Marijuana smoking		ciprofloxacin
		allopurinol
Phenytoin therapy	Cirrhosis	
	Cardiac failure	
Rifampicin therapy	Sustained fever	
	Old age	
Alcohol	Influenza vaccination	
	Oral contraceptives	

Fig. 2.25 Factors affecting the metabolism of theophylline.

attacks have not been borne out by moderately large studies carried out over 6–12 months.

Long-acting bronchodilators should be given only to patients already receiving regular anti-inflammatory agents, such as inhaled steroids. The regular inhaled steroids should be continued with the long-acting bronchodilators, and short-acting bronchodilators should also be used as necessary.

Increasing the inhaled steroid or adding the long-acting inhaled β_2-agonist are alternative steps at this point. The next step is to combine these two treatments.

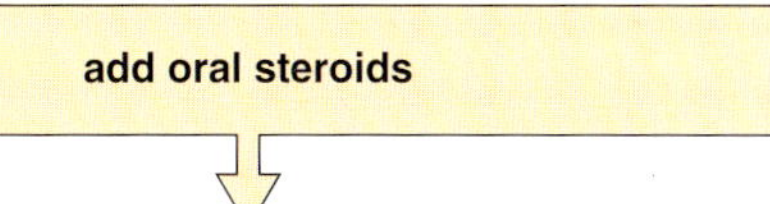

Oral steroids have many side-effects (**Figs 2.26 & 2.27**). They should, therefore, be reserved for asthmatic patients with persistent problems despite full inhaled therapy, whose compliance and inhaler technique has been assessed and optimized. Before embarking on oral steroids it is also worth reviewing the question of continuing exposure to precipitating factors.

Adverse effects of oral steroid treatment	
Growth retardation in children	Amenorrhoea
Truncal obesity	Hyperglycaemia
Hypertension	Hyperlipidaemia
Osteoporosis	Hypokalaemia
Aseptic bone necrosis (femoral head)	Mood change
Proximal myopathy	Sleep disturbance
Cataracts	Steroid psychosis
Poor wound healing	Haemorrhage from peptic ulcers
Immunosuppression	

Fig. 2.26 Adverse effects of oral steroid treatment.

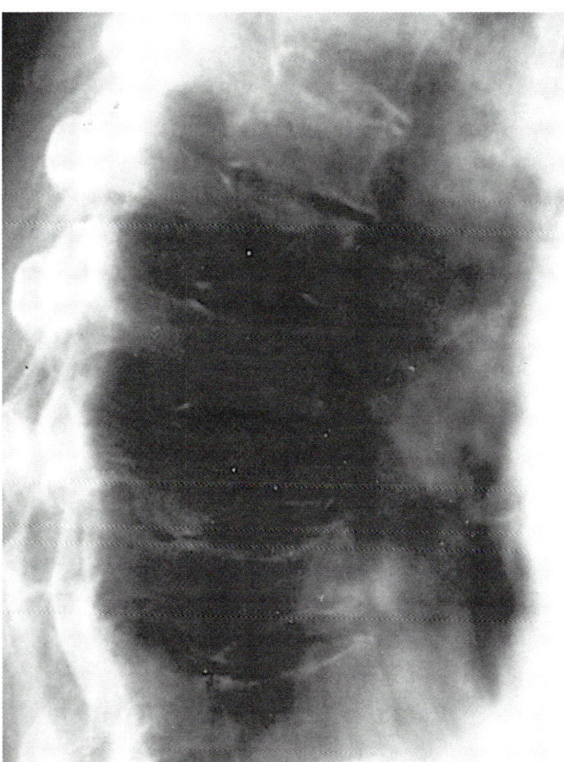

Fig. 2.27 Osteoporosis leading to vertebral collapse in a patient with asthma who had received long-term oral steroid therapy. This radiograph shows severe osteoporosis with early wedging of vertebral bodies in the mid-thoracic region. Episodes of vertebral collapse are painful, and result in progressive kyphosis. Osteoporosis also makes the patient more susceptible to fractures at the hip, wrist and elsewhere.

Initially, a short course of oral steroids should be prescribed to re-establish control, which can usually be subsequently maintained with inhaled steroids (**Fig. 2.28**). Short courses of oral steroids are frequently used for exacerbations of asthma. Adverse effects are rare, but include increased appetite, restlessness and sleep disturbance, gastro-intestinal upset and, occasionally, frank psychotic effects.

If a decision is made to maintain oral therapy then inhaled steroids should be continued, so that the oral dose is minimized. Nebulized budesonide may be used to avoid or limit the use of oral steroids in some patients who have not responded adequately to other forms of inhaled steroid.

therapeutic alternatives

Continuous subcutaneous infusion of a β_2-agonist is used occasionally for patients with repeated attacks, or for 'brittle asthma' in which there are wide swings in peak flow with no particular pattern (**Fig. 2.29**). High tissue levels are obtained with this method. The site of the subcutaneous infusion is changed by the patient or a nurse every 2–3 days (**Fig. 2.30**). A very small proportion of patients are resistant to the effects of steroids and may need high beta-2-agonist doses. It is important to recognise steroid resistance so that the drugs are not continued unnecessarily.

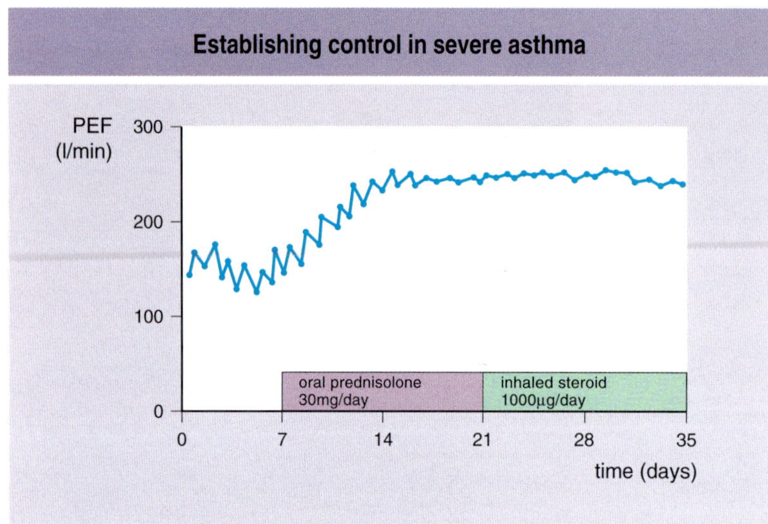

Fig. 2.28 Establishing control in severe asthma. A short course of oral steroid therapy may be helpful in establishing or re-establishing control of severe asthma, but the patient should be weaned on to inhaled steroid therapy, which usually allows continued good control.

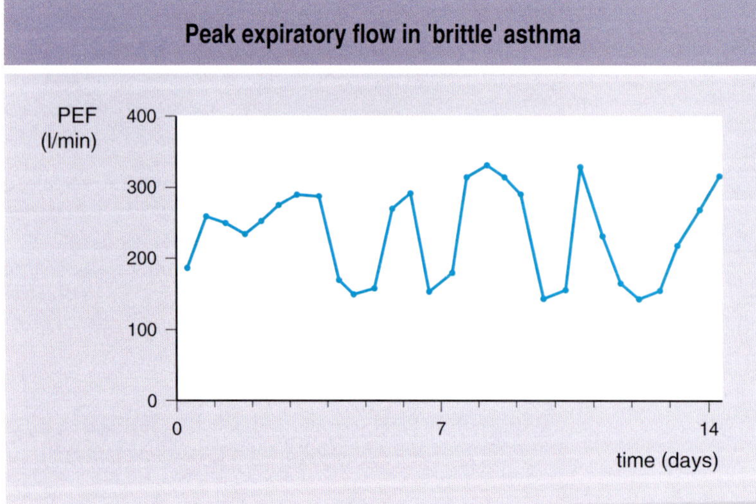

Fig. 2.29 Peak expiratory flow in 'brittle' asthma. There are wide variations in PEF, and the patient had frequent acute exacerbations without any warning features. This type of asthma may require treatment with regular long-acting β_2-agonist therapy or by continuous subcutaneous infusion of a short-acting β_2-agonist.

Methotrexate can be used in a weekly oral dose to reduce the oral steroid dose where high doses are needed for asthma control. The effects of methotrexate take several months to appear. Side-effects include bone marrow suppression, liver toxicity and pulmonary fibrosis. The blood picture and liver function tests need to be monitored throughout treatment.

Cyclosporin A has helped chronic, difficult-to-control asthma in some trials. Blood levels must be monitored and the main toxic effects are on the kidney.

Leukotriene antagonists, and other drugs which act on various parts of the pathway of arachidonic acid metabolism, are becoming available (**Fig. 2.31**). It is hoped that they will have an anti-inflammatory action without the potentially deleterious effects of steroids, which act as global suppressors of inflammation. Their place in asthma treatment should be defined over the next few years.

Antihistamines have no significant direct effects in asthma, but they may have a role in the management of associated rhinitis. Control of rhinitis with antihistamines or topical nasal steroid therapy is often associated with decreased airway hyperresponsiveness and improved control of asthma – especially where the asthma has an obvious allergic basis.

Alternative therapies, such as homeopathy, yoga, and acupuncture, are tried by at least 25% of most asthmatic populations, reflecting concern over the possible toxicity of conventional treatments. Few of these methods have been assessed in controlled clinical trials.

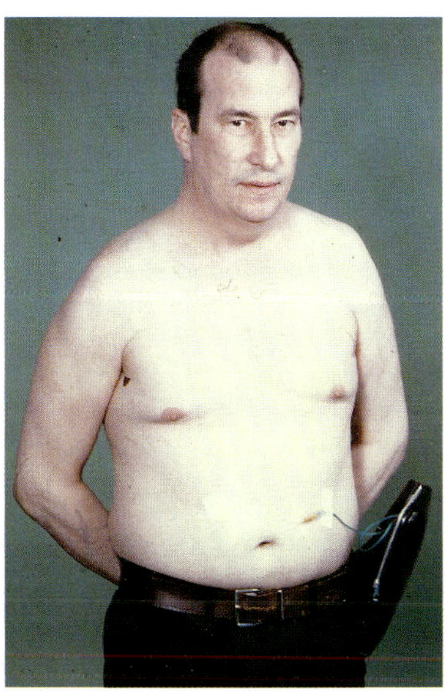

Fig. 2.30 A patient with severe 'brittle' asthma receiving continuous subcutaneous β_2-agonist via a small battery-driven syringe pump. A very few patients may be dramatically helped by continuous subcutaneous selective β_2-agonist infusion. This patient varied the dose in a similar fashion to a diabetic between day and night and his morning PEF dips were stopped.

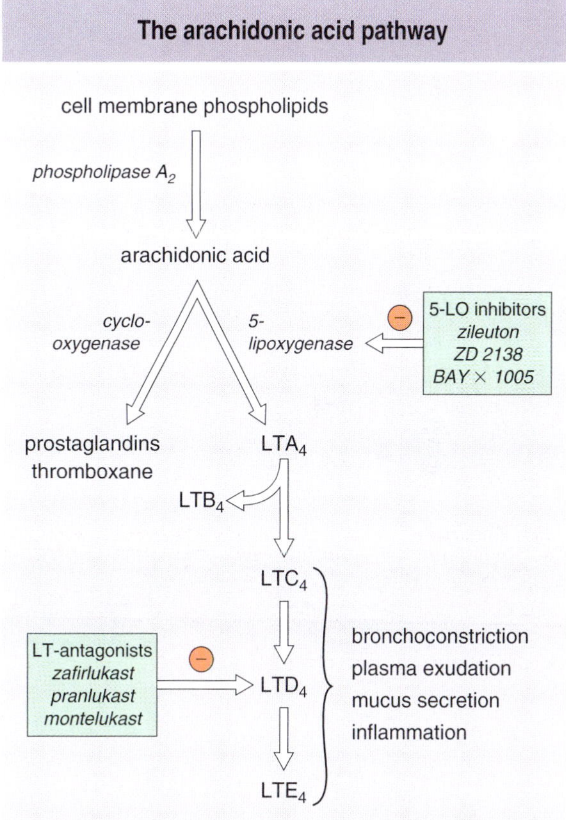

Fig. 2.31 The arachidonic acid pathway and the site of action of leukotriene antagonists and 5-lipoxygenase inhibitors.

Stepping up and stepping down

Treatment does not always begin at the first level of the management algorithm. For example, if a patient presents with persistent or severe symptoms then occasional use of a β_2-agonist is not an adequate treatment. Entry to the algorithm should therefore be at a level likely to allow control of the disease. In some cases this may mean starting with a course of oral steroids. It may be better to begin with a moderately 'aggressive' approach and ease back to a lesser level of treatment for regular control (**Fig. 2.32**).

Where the initial treatment is aggressive, stepping down can be done quite soon after control is established. Where the starting treatment is moderate, stepping down should be more gradual. This is particularly important with anti-inflammatory treatments which, once initiated, should be continued with good control for 6 months or more. Once the treatment has been reduced or stopped, patients should be observed carefully for a return of symptoms, which would prompt the reinstatement of higher dose therapy.

Patients may enter a state of apparent remission after withdrawal of inhaled steroids. However, they should always be considered at risk of further severe asthma should the right provocation arise, since inflammatory changes in the airways are likely to persist.

Continued education of the patient in the recognition and management of recurrences or exacerbations is essential.

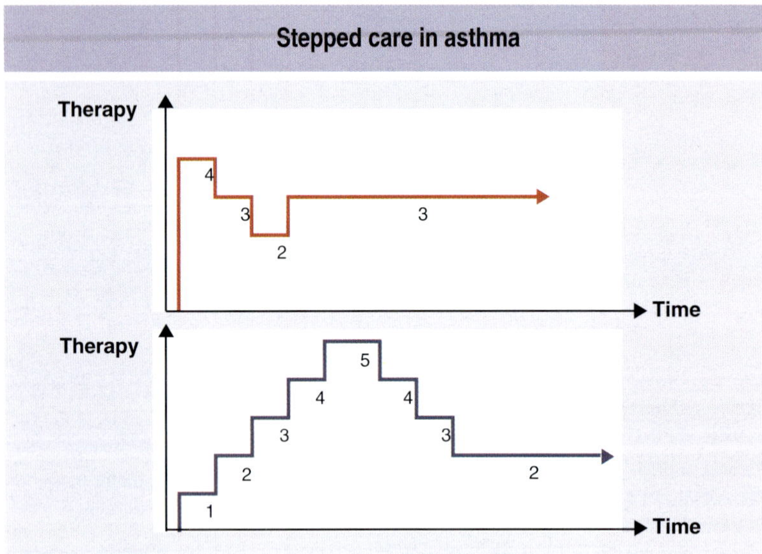

Fig. 2.32 Stepped care in asthma. Starting treatment at a higher entry (upper figure) may give faster, easier control than a gradual increase through all the steps of treatment (lower figure).

Deaths from asthma are rare in children, numbering 40–45 each year in England and Wales. Predisposing factors for death in children are similar to those in adults and include delayed treatment and severe bronchial hyperresponsiveness. However, there is evidence that although most asthma deaths in children could be prevented, a small proportion may be entirely unpredictable and therefore unavoidable.

history and clinical presentation

The classic presentation of asthma in childhood is with paroxysmal coughing, wheezing, a sensation of tightness in the chest, and breathlessness. These symptoms may be exacerbated by an intercurrent viral infection, by factors such as exercise or sudden exposure to the cold, by exposure to allergens such as house dust mite or pollen, or by exposure to irritants such as cigarette smoke or exhaust fumes.

The severity of the condition may be judged by its effects on daily life, such as sleep, school and sports, as well as by the frequency and severity of the symptoms.

signs and symptoms

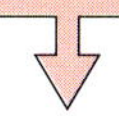

Children presenting with suspected asthma will sometimes have the stigmata of allergy, such as rhinitis (*see* Chapter 1 – in fact 80–85% of asthmatic children have allergic rhinitis), atopic eczema (*see* Chapter 7), swollen eyelids (**Fig. 3.2**), nose rubbing, or mouth breathing (*see* Chapter 1). Otitis media and allergic conjunctivitis are also frequently associated with asthma.

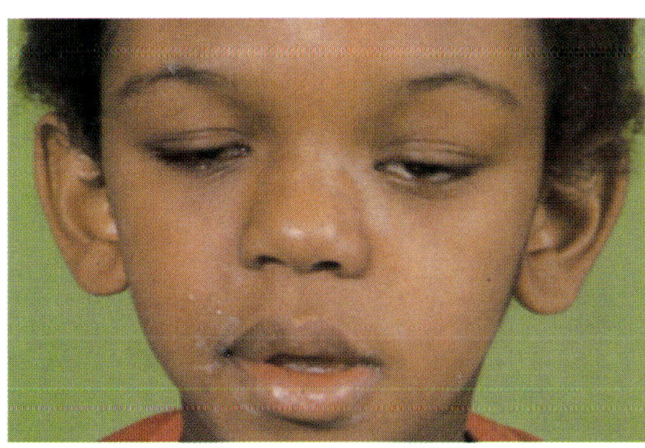

Fig. 3.2 A 7-year-old boy with asthma. Although asthma was his major clinical problem, he has characteristic atopic facies, with a lethargic expression, infraorbital and perioral oedema, a swollen and congested nose and some facial eczema, especially around the mouth.

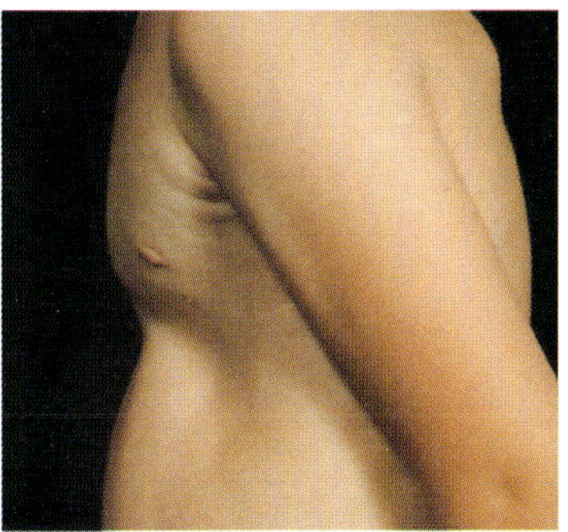

Fig. 3.3 Pigeon chest (pectus carinatum) in a 10-year-old girl with asthma. Her asthma had been poorly controlled throughout childhood. The sternum and costochondral junctions form a prominent ridge in the anterior chest, and the ribs slope away steeply to either side. Pigeon chest is usually a manifestation of the impact of chronic hyperinflation of the chest on growth in childhood.

3 Childhood Asthma

Anthony D Milner

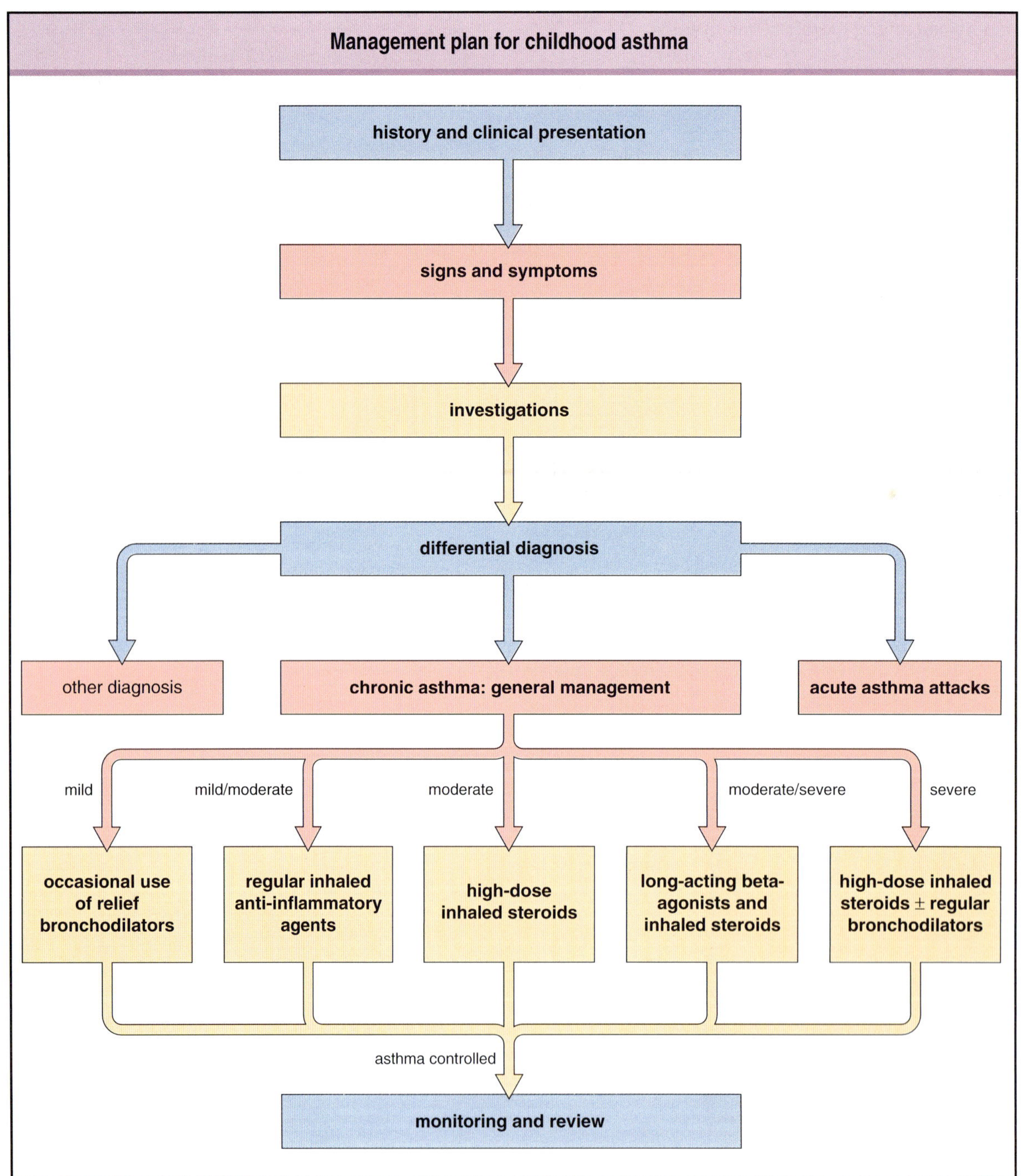

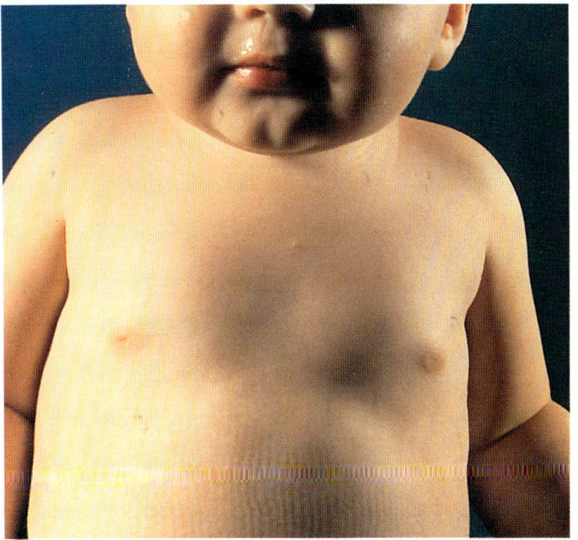

Fig. 3.4 Harrison's sulci in an infant with previously undiagnosed asthma. The sulci are horizontal grooves on each side of the chest, several rib spaces wide. They are thought to occur as a result of the traction of the diaphragms on the lower ribs during episodes of wheezing.

Chronic asthma, particularly when untreated, can result in a number of chest wall deformities including funnel chest, pigeon chest (**Fig. 3.3**), and Harrison's sulci (**Fig. 3.4**).

Children with severe chronic asthma may also demonstrate abnormally low growth compared to that of their more healthy peers. Although this is likely to be most often seen in untreated patients, it can also occur where the asthma is poorly managed. For this reason, it is important to make regular, accurate measurements of height and weight for plotting on centile charts (**Fig. 3.5**).

investigations

A chest radiograph is needed to exclude other diagnoses when symptoms are persistent. Most children with asthma have chest films that are either normal or show only non-specific changes (**Fig. 3.6**).

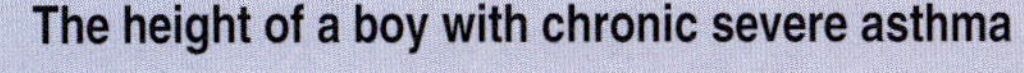

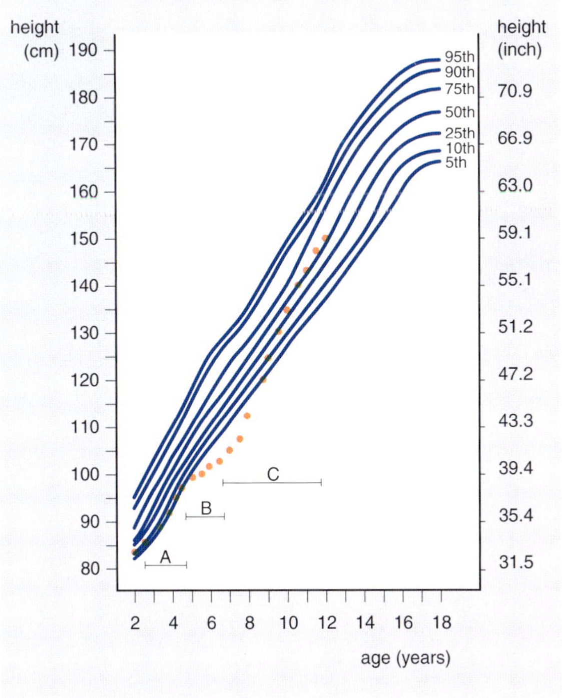

Fig. 3.5 The height of a boy with chronic severe asthma, plotted on a height centile chart for boys. When first diagnosed the child was on the 10th centile (A). His uncontrolled asthma was subsequently treated with a prolonged course of oral prednisolone therapy, during which his growth was significantly impaired (B). Later he was weaned onto inhaled steroid therapy while maintaining control of his asthma (C). At this stage catch-up growth was seen, and he reached the 50th centile.

3 Childhood Asthma

Anthony D Milner

Introduction

Asthma is the most common chronic disease of childhood. The prevalence is 10–16% in the UK, and is even higher in some other countries, reaching 25% in Australia, for example. Admission rates to hospital have also increased over recent years, particularly for infants. Factors such as increased diagnostic awareness may be important here, but underlying increases in morbidity in this age group cannot be ruled out.

Although asthma responds well to treatment, this disease is both underdiagnosed and undertreated. One study in the UK found that less than half of all cases of childhood asthma were correctly identified and treated (**Fig. 3.1**). Undiagnosed asthma in children is associated with significant limitations on the child's everyday activities and a higher than normal number of lost school days. This can have a serious impact on the child's social and academic progress. In addition, there is the danger of delayed development and acute asthma attacks, which can be severe or even life threatening.

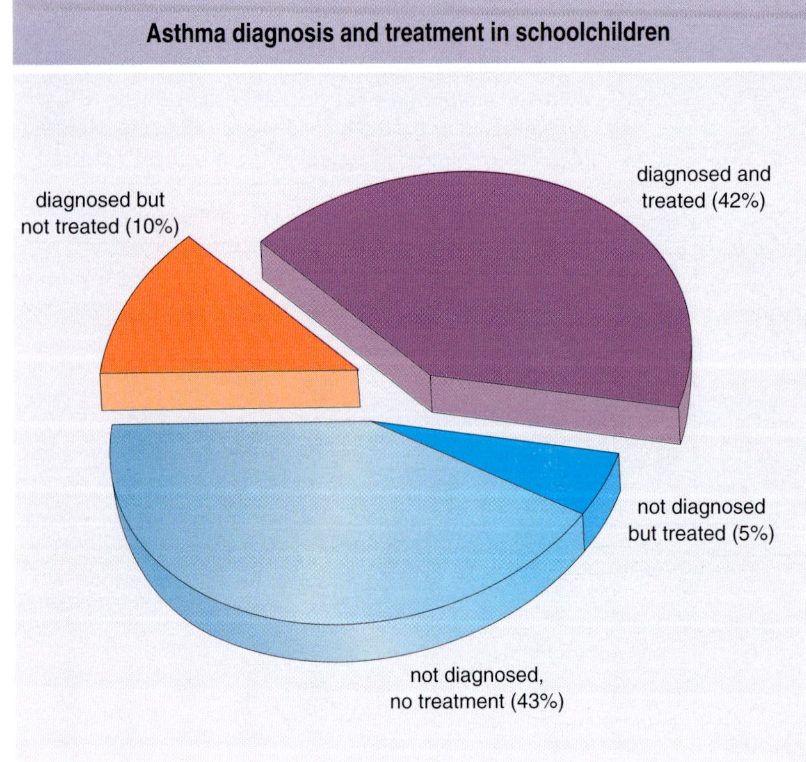

Fig. 3.1 Asthma diagnosis and treatment in schoolchildren. A study in Nottingham (UK) showed an overall prevalence of asthma of 12%. Of these children, nearly half remained undiagnosed, and just 42% were both diagnosed and treated. (Data from Hill *et al.*, *Arch Dis Child* 1989;64:246.)

therapy is the only alternative. This is normally administered by a jet nebulizer (**Figs 3.17 & 3.18**). (Ultrasonic nebulizers can also be used for drugs in solution, but are unsuitable for the delivery of particulate suspensions, such as budesonide.) A driving flow of air or oxygen (in acute asthma), at a rate of at least 6 L/min, is required for optimum use. Speed of nebulization is particularly important in this age-group, as treatments lasting longer than 10 minutes are unlikely to be completed. Most anti-asthma drugs are available in a form suitable for nebulizing, but budesonide is the only effectively nebulizable steroid.

Children between 18 months old and school age are best treated with a pMDI via a valved spacer device and facemask or (preferably) a mouthpiece (**Fig. 3.19**). By the age of 33 months, most can use a mouthpiece. The most important advantage of these devices is that there is no need to coordinate inhalation with actuation of the inhaler. The spacer also allows time for the propellant to evaporate from the particles, so that they are both smaller and slower when they reach the upper airway. This improves delivery to the lower airways by as much as 50%, compared with pMDIs used without spacers.

Children over 4 years old can be trained to use almost any pMDI with a spacer device or any dry powder inhaler. For children up to the age of 10 years, dry powder inhalers (**Figs 3.20 & 3.21**) are preferable to pMDIs without spacers as they require less coordination.

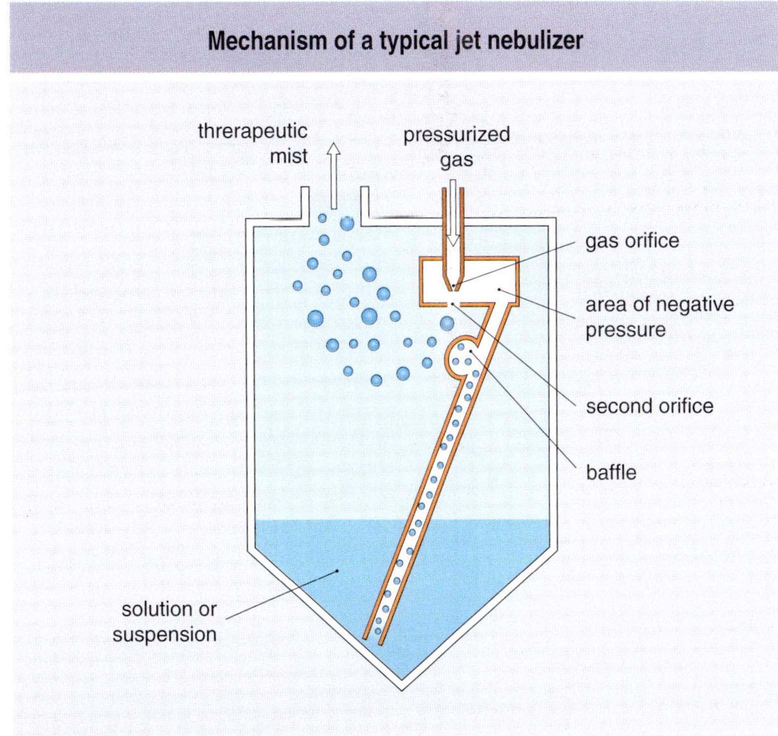

Fig. 3.17 Mechanism of a typical jet nebulizer. The pressurized air or oxygen enters the nebulizer chamber via a fine tube with a narrow orifice, and the jet creates a venturi effect. This sucks droplets of the drug solution or suspension up another tube where it hits a baffle and is broken up into a very fine particulate aerosol. This therapeutic mist leaves the chamber and is inhaled by the patient.

Parents who smoke should be strongly encouraged to stop. Ideally the house should be made a tobacco smoke-free zone.

Pets should be excluded from the home. If this can't be done, then they should at least be excluded from the child's bedroom. Regular washing of cats can reduce levels of cat antigen in the fur, but is an imperfect solution to the problem.

Exposure to dust mite antigen can be reduced by control measures (*see* Chapter 1).

The importance of correct treatment

It is very important that both the child and his/her caregivers are able to treat and monitor the progress of the disease, as inadequate suppression of inflammation can precipitate acute episodes (see below). It also encourages the development of structural changes, such as fibrosis and smooth muscle hypertrophy, which narrow airways and make the disease more resistant to treatment.

Inhalation devices (described below) must be used correctly to obtain the full benefit of the drug that they dispense. Incorrect use means that the disease is undertreated and progression to a more severe form is encouraged.

It is also important that both child and carer fully appreciate the difference between prophylactic and relief therapy. Failure to make this distinction may lead to overuse of beta-agonists, a practice that has been associated (controversially) with an increased risk of death.

Inhalation devices

Inhalation devices allow drugs to be delivered direct to the site of action. Inhaled therapy offers many advantages: onset of action is rapid, the dose administered is relatively small, and the risk of systemic side-effects is low. To be fully effective, inhalation devices must be correctly operated, and this can be a problem when the user is a child, particularly a very young child. The range of commonly available inhalation devices for children is listed in **Figure 3.15**.

The first option for treating infants younger than 18 months is to use a pMDI with spacer and face mask (**Fig. 3.16**). If this is not tolerated, nebulized inhalation

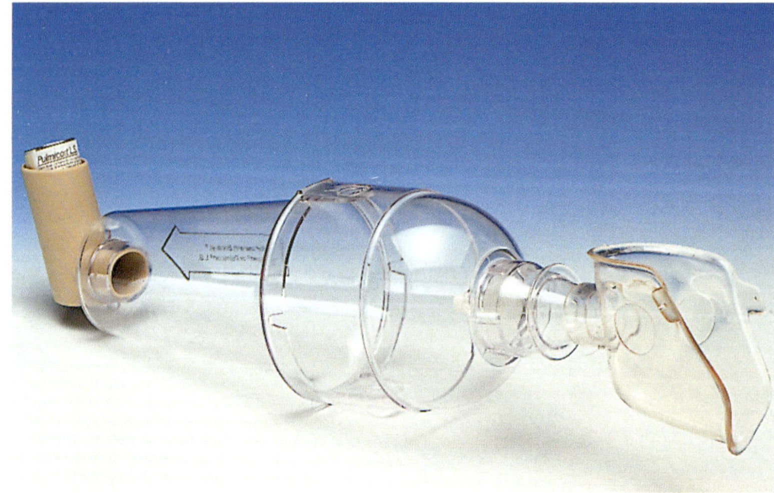

Fig. 3.16 A large volume spacer device fitted with a face mask. The relative portability of the spacer makes administration of medication much simpler to arrange than with a nebulizer. The valve is removed from the spacer device when the face mask is fitted so that the infant simply breathes in and out of the spacer for a short period of time while therapy is administered. Many small and large volume spacer devices are available, but it is important to use a combination of drug, pMDI, spacer and mask which have been designed for compatibility.

chronic asthma: general management

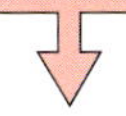

The aims of management

Management of asthma in childhood aims to resolve acute symptoms, and then to reduce the risk of long-term morbidity by the early use of anti-inflammatory agents. A successful outcome is measured by the minimal impact of the controlled disease on the child's life: there is no waking at night, few symptoms during the day, no interruption of school, no restriction on leisure activities or sport, and infrequent need for beta-agonist relief.

Environmental factors

The first step is to avoid or remove precipitating factors. This means reducing exposure to everyday environmental allergens, such as house dust mite and animal dander, and reducing levels of irritants such as cigarette smoke and exhaust fumes.

Inhalation devices in the treatment of childhood asthma

Age (years)	Inhalation device	Relieving treatment	Preventive treatment
<2	Nebulizer and air compressor or valved spacer and face mask	Salbutamol Terbutaline Ipratropium bromide	Sodium cromoglycate Budesonide
2–4	Metered dose inhaler with valved spacer		
	Nebuhaler	Terbutaline	Budesonide
	Volumatic	Salbutamol	BDP
	Aerochamber	Ipratropium bromide	–
	Fisonair	–	Sodium cromoglycate
	Nebulizer for acute episodes		
5–8	Powder inhalers		
	Spinhaler	–	Sodium cromoglycate
	Diskhaler	Salbutamol	BDP, fluticasone
	Rotahaler	Salbutamol	BDP
	Diskus/Accuhaler	Salmeterol	Fluticasone
	Turbuhaler/Turbohaler	Terbutaline, salbutamol	Budesonide
	Metered dose inhaler with valved spacer for acute attacks instead of nebulizer	All of the above	High dose inhaled steroids
>8	Autohaler	Salbutamol	Sodium cromoglycate, BDP
	Metered dose inhaler *with training*, or powder inhalers	All of the above	All of the above

Fig. 3.15 Inhalation devices in the treatment of childhood asthma. The suitability of devices depends upon the age of the child, and on the degree of cooperation that they offer. (Modified from Warner *et al.*, *Arch Dis Child* 1992;**67**:240–248.)

An acute severe attack of asthma indicates that the chronic management of the disease is inadequate. A full review of the child's management plan should be carried out, with special attention paid to the adequacy of the anti-inflammatory therapy, and the likely level of compliance with that therapy.

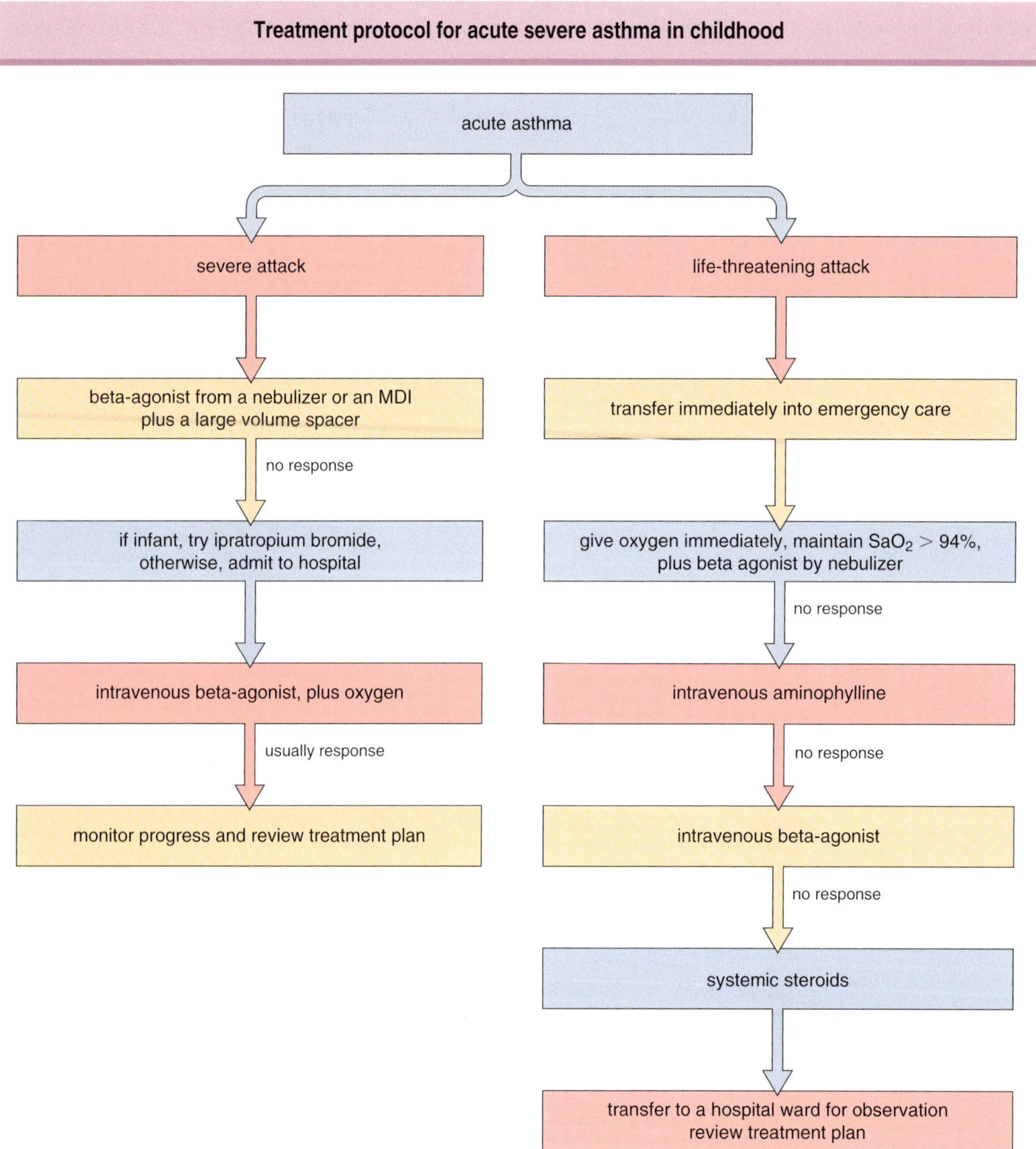

Fig. 3.14 Treatment protocol for acute severe asthma in childhood.

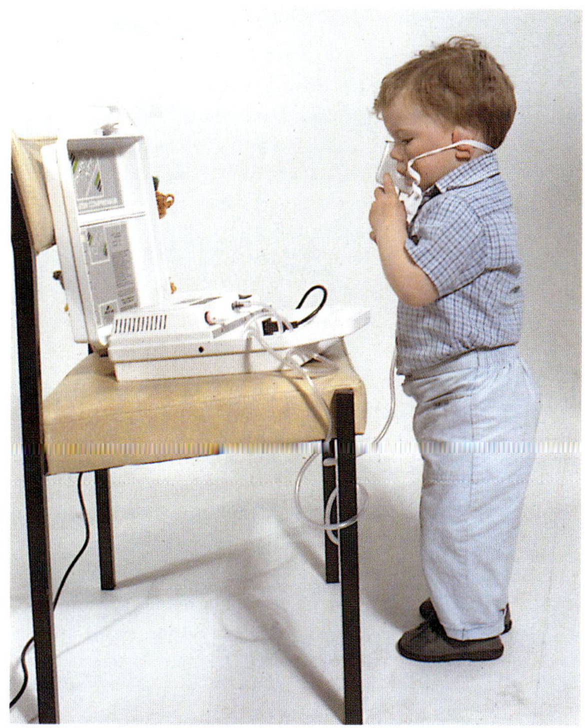

Fig. 3.18 A two-year-old child using a nebulizer system for his prophylactic asthma medication. The air compressor is on the chair and the nebulizer chamber is in his hand. Most powerful compressors need mains electricity, but foot-pump operated models are also available. This child is using a face mask, but mouthpiece inhalation is preferable, as it minimizes the risk of local side-effects.

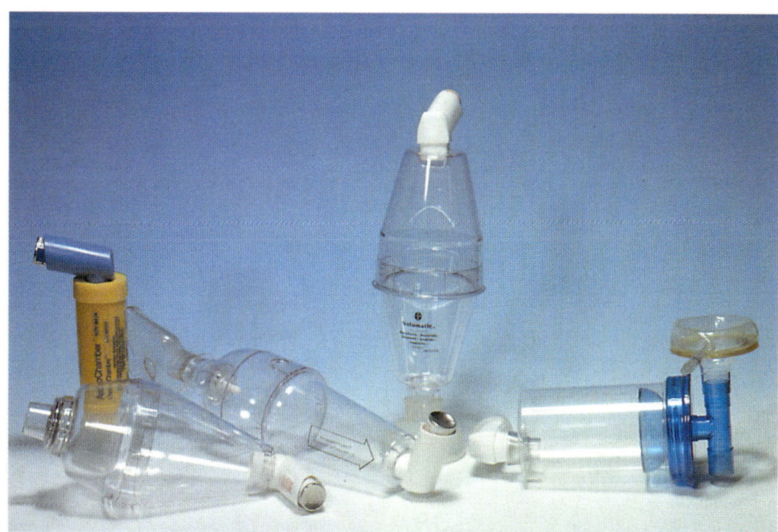

Fig. 3.19 Various forms of spacer device for the inhalation of drugs from metered dose inhalers. All these devices allow some evaporation of propellant and slowing of particles, which enhances lung deposition and lessens impaction of particles in the oropharynx. The large volume spacers allow good delivery even in the absence of co-ordinated inhalation and actuation. They also have a valve, which permits expiration during use, and are the most suitable devices for children below the age of five years.

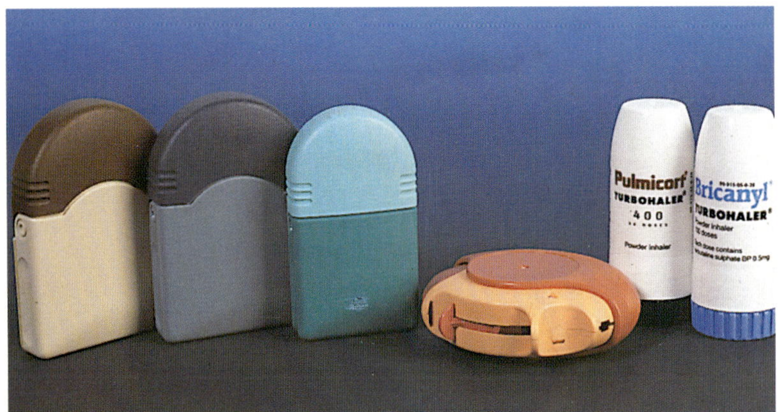

Fig. 3.20 Some modern dry powder inhalers. Two examples of the 8-dose Diskhaler (left), a 4-dose Diskhaler (centre), a Diskus (Accuhaler) and two examples of the Turbuhaler (Turbohaler). Diskus and Turbuhaler are true multidose inhalers.

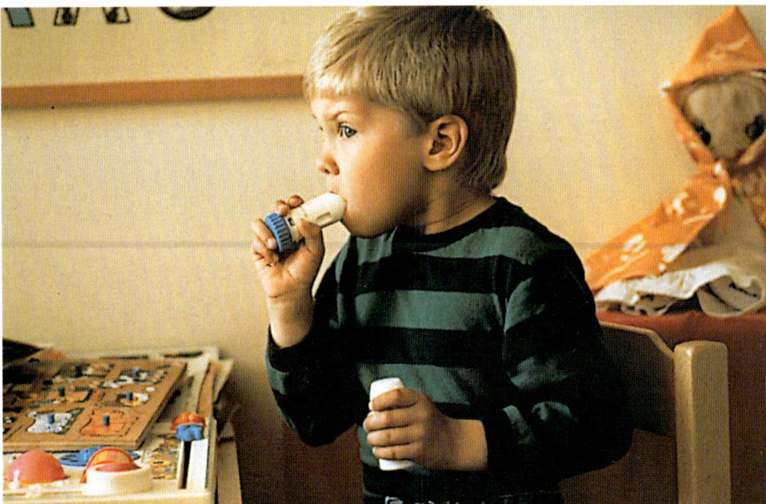

Fig. 3.21 A dry powder inhaler in use. This is a Turbuhaler (Turbohaler), here used to deliver dry powder terbutaline. Most children over the age of five years can master the technique of using dry powder inhalers, and sometimes much younger children can also do so.

Pressurized metered dose inhalers without spacers can be used by many older children (**Figs 3.22 & 3.23**). Although optimum use requires both skill and coordination (which must be checked), pMDIs are often the lowest cost portable inhalation devices available.

The five-step management plan

Inhalation devices form the first line of treatment at all stages of the five-step treatment plan for chronic asthma, outlined below. Treatment should enter this plan at the treatment level most appropriate to the severity of their condition.

Before treatment is stepped up it is vital to ensure that the current level of therapy is being correctly administered: the child should be using an inhaler appropriate to his/her age, the technique should be good, and the parents should understand the principles of effective management.

If after a few months of therapy the symptoms are minimal, a reduction in therapy may be possible. A diary card, to record peak flow measurements, may be helpful in the period before and after the step down.

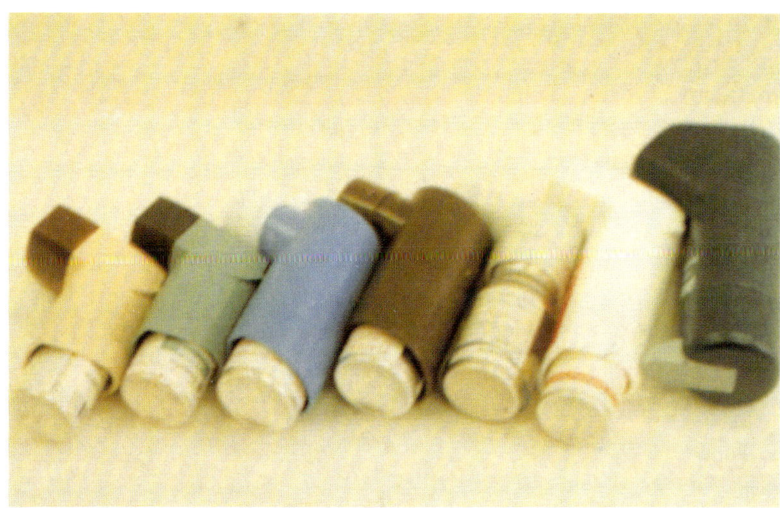

Fig. 3.22 A selection of pMDIs. All inhaled drugs are available in this form. On the right is an autohaler, in which a spring-loaded device actuates the inhaler only when air is drawn through, thus overcoming some of the co-ordination problems which may otherwise occur with these inhalers.

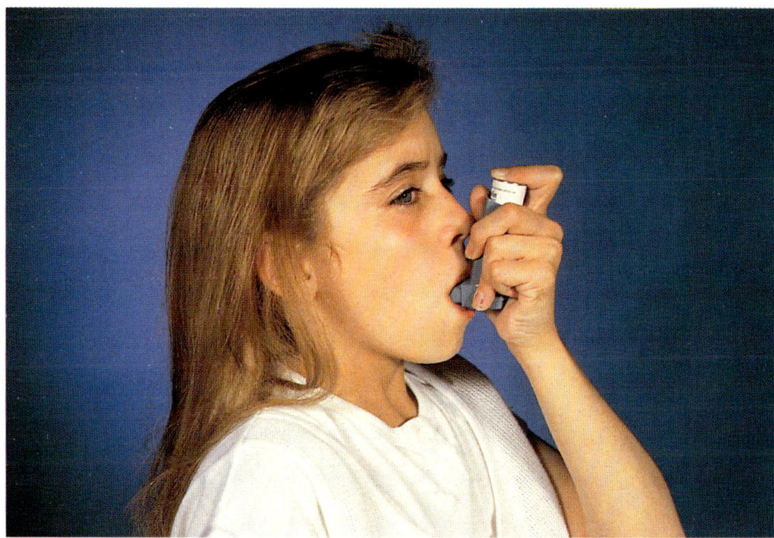

Fig. 3.23 A child using a pMDI. It is essential that children are educated in the correct use of all inhalers, and the need for coordination between inspiration and actuation often leads to particular problems for those who use pMDIs. The supervising physician and/or asthma nurse specialist should always observe the child's use of the device, and arrange further training if necessary.

occasional use of relief bronchodilators

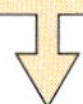

Short acting beta-agonists are taken 'as required' for symptom relief. Inhaled drugs should be used wherever possible, as bronchodilator syrups are much less effective than inhaled beta-agonists and have more systemic side-effects. If treatment is required more regularly than once daily, the child should advance to the next step in treatment.

regular inhaled anti-inflammatory agents

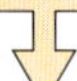

Intermittent inhaled short-acting beta-agonists are given as required. In addition, sodium cromoglycate (cromolyn) is given as powder (20 mg tid) or via metered dose inhaler and large volume spacer (10 mg tid). Cromoglycate is safe and seems helpful in many children; it is still recommended as first-line preventive treatment in some paediatric guidelines. A therapeutic trial for 4–6 weeks is indicated before the child progresses to the next treatment level. An age-appropriate delivery system should be used, and a peak flow meter should be supplied where appropriate.

long acting beta-agonists and inhaled steroids

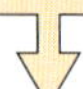

The patient is given inhaled short-acting beta-agonists as required, and also receives beclomethasone or budesonide 50–200 µg bd. A five day course of soluble prednisolone 1–2 mg/kg/day, or a temporary increase (double dose) of inhaled steroids can be given for stabilization. After one month, the effect on symptoms and/or peak flow measurements is assessed, and the dose is adjusted accordingly.

Metered dose inhalers must be used with a spacer, to increase lung deposition and minimize oropharyngeal deposition. If a pMDI without spacer or a dry powder inhaler is used, children should be taught to either rinse or brush their teeth following each dose, to reduce absorption of steroid deposited in the mouth.

If the control of the asthma symptoms remains inadequate, regular, twice-daily dosing with a long-acting, inhaled beta-agonist may also be useful. These drugs produce bronchodilatation in children for up to 12 hours, inhibit exercise-induced bronchoconstriction, and protect against methacholine challenge for a similar length of time. The long-term clinical effects of these drugs have yet to be determined, and they should be reserved for use as a supplementary treatment in children already receiving anti-inflammatory drugs.

high-dose inhaled steroids

Inhaled short-acting beta-agonists are given as required, together with beclomethasone or budesonide 400–800 µg daily via a large volume spacer or dry powder device. For additional control, a short course of prednisolone can be considered.

high-dose inhaled steroids and bronchodilators

Where attacks are frequent, or where there are significant effects on daily life, higher doses of inhaled steroids are needed. Inhaled steroids (800 µg daily) should be added to existing treatments, together with sustained-release xanthines or nebulized beta-agonists. Oral steroid therapy should very rarely be necessary in childhood asthma, and can sometimes be avoided by the use of nebulized steroid (budesonide). Sustained release xanthines produce effective bronchodilatation but have appreciable side effects (gastrointestinal disorders, sleep disturbance, and psychological changes) in up to one-third of children. Thus, although they may be helpful, particularly for nocturnal symptoms, monitoring of serum or salivary concentrations is recommended. Similar clinical improvements have been shown with sustained release preparations of salbutamol, a treatment with far fewer side-effects.

monitoring and review

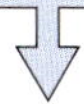

This can be done by the older child or carer, as well as the doctor, by the noting of symptoms and regular measurement of PEFR with the peak flow meter. The medication is then stepped up or down as necessary. Regular anti-inflammatory treatment can sometimes be stopped after 6-12 months of few or no symptoms but objective monitoring of airway function should be continued initially, and treatment re-started if there is a deterioration. If treatment is failing, check compliance and correct use of devices.

the normal self-administered treatments. The episode may either be very acute, with symptoms developing over minutes or hours, or may be more gradual, developing over a period of days. The breathlessness and wheeze are associated with reduced lung function, which is measurable with a peak flow meter or by spirometry. Because symptoms are so variable, the peak expiratory flow (PEF) measurements are often the best and most objective way for professionals to characterise an attack in a patient.

Acute attacks in adults and children over five years of age are very similar. Children tend to present with shorter histories and recover faster than adults.

In children under five years the diagnosis is less clear cut, owing to diagnostic overlap with viral bronchiolitis. Measurements are difficult and treatment [illegible] different.

This section deals principally with the treatment of adults, although most of it is also applicable to the 5–16-year old, with some dose adjustment. Diagnosis and treatment of the under-fives is considered in Chapter 3.

Causes of acute severe asthma

Although most asthma probably has an allergic basis, finding a specific cause for individual episodes of acute severe asthma is rarely possible. There are many well-documented trigger factors but their effects can vary hugely between individuals. The allergic reaction can be rapid with symptoms of wheeze and breathlessness developing within 15 minutes of exposure. These are probably Type I hypersensitivity reactions, mediated by IgE. The mechanism is similar to the dermal response to a skin prick test (*see* **Figs 1.22 & 1.23**) About 30% of Europeans have one or more positive skin prick tests to common allergens, and most asthma occurs within this atopic part of the population. In addition, many asthmatics have a second, IgG mediated late reaction which commences typically 6–8 hours after exposure. This reaction may persist for many hours and is probably more important in causing airway inflammation (*see* **Fig. 2.7**).

Possible causes of an acute episode may include an acute viral infection (**Fig. 4.2**) superimposed on a

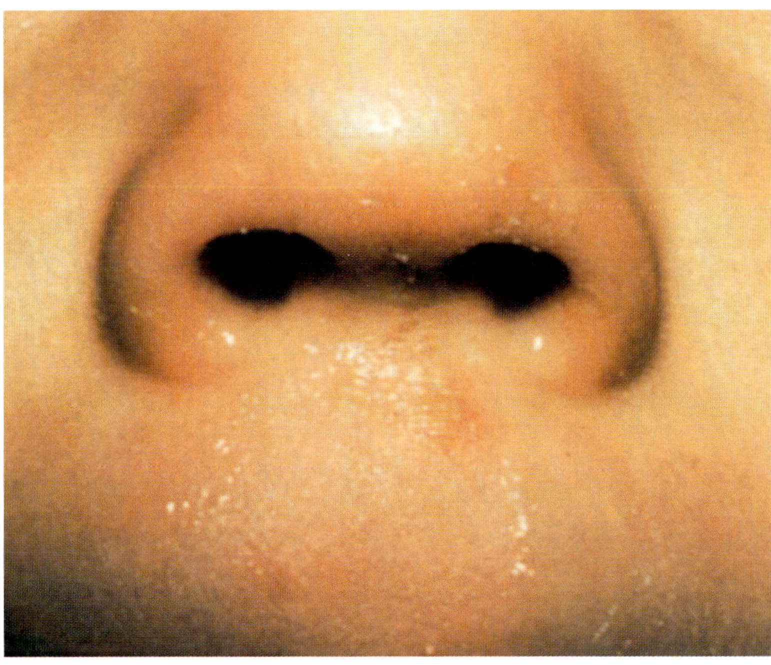

Fig. 4.2 Acute viral infections may precipitate acute severe asthma in susceptible individuals. Upper respiratory tract infections, including the common cold, are frequent triggers of acute attacks, especially in children.

4 Acute Severe Asthma

Michael G Pearson

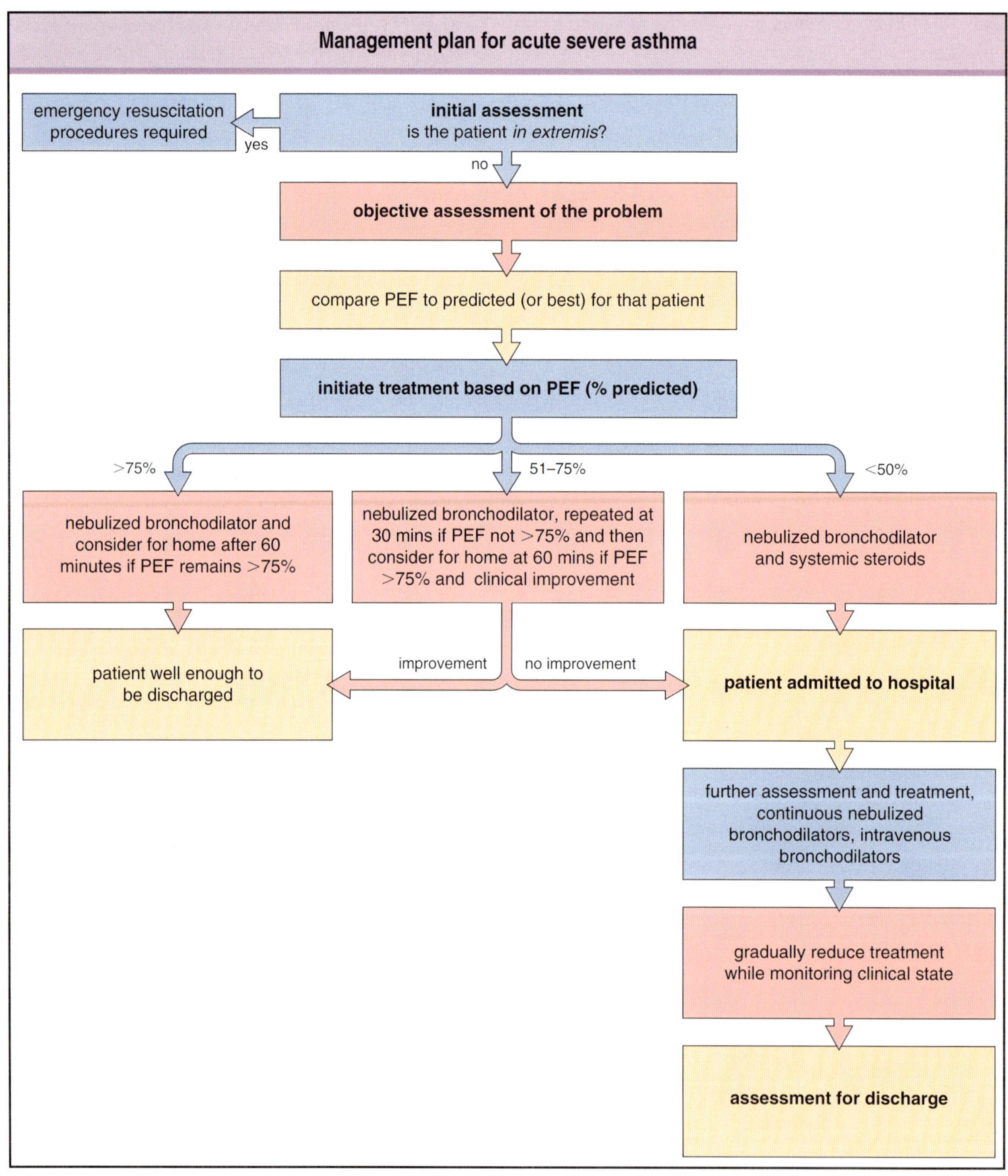

chronic low-grade reaction to house dust mite or a pet. Less commonly, it may be an acute response to a substance at work, such as isocyanate in spray paints (**Fig. 4.3**), to moulds in the home disturbed during cleaning, or even to a food product, such as tartrazine (E102). When specific causes are found, discussions with the patient are needed, to determine whether avoidance is a practical possibility.

Pathology

There are two components to acute severe asthma: bronchospasm and inflammation (*see also* Chapter 2). The inflammatory reaction is associated with a cellular infiltrate into the intimal layers and exudation into the airway lumen. The luminal secretions are thicker and more viscid than normal and can aggregate to form 'mucous

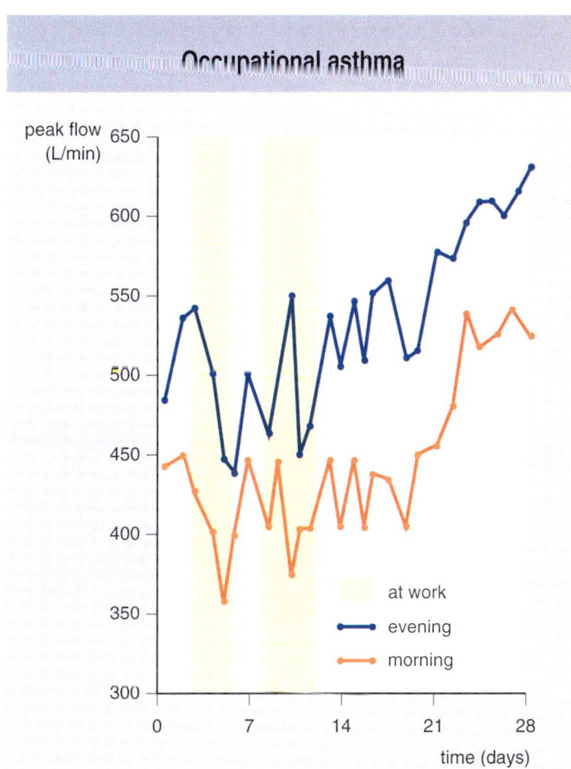

Fig. 4.3 Occupational exposure may provoke acute severe asthma. PEF monitoring in this patient who worked as a paint sprayer showed low PEF values during work periods. Values improved at weekends and, more markedly, during a 2-week holiday. The patient was allergic to isocyanate, a common provoking substance found in spray paints.

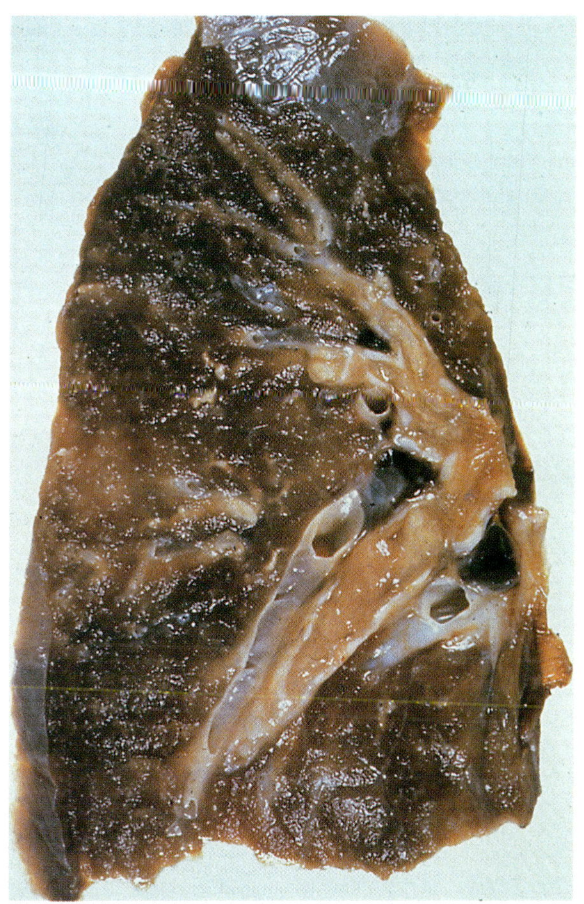

Fig. 4.4 A section through the lung in a case of fatal asthma. Note the extensive mucous plugging of the intrapulmonary airways.

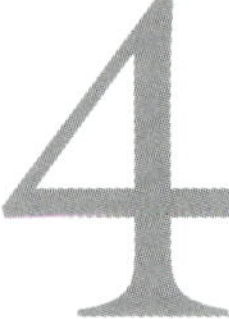

4 Acute Severe Asthma

Michael G Pearson

Asthma varies from a mild condition, causing a little wheezing on exertion but no significant disability, to a severe chronic disabling state leading to respiratory failure and death. At any stage of the chronic stable state, asthma can deteriorate acutely, and it is these acute flare-ups which constitute acute severe asthma. More detail of the aetiology and allergic basis of asthma appear in Chapters 1 and 2.

Deaths due to asthma are a cause for concern in many countries because of the relatively large numbers involved (**Fig. 4.1**), and because studies indicate that about 60% of these deaths could have been prevented.

What is acute asthma?

Asthma is a very variable condition and there is no single definition of an 'acute severe attack'. Uncomfortable attacks of mild-to-moderate bronchospasm, which resolve either spontaneously or with short-acting bronchodilators, are a common feature of chronic asthma that most patients learn to cope with and accept as part of their condition.

Acute severe asthma is characterized by a more marked degree of bronchospasm. The patient becomes distressed and is unable to control the symptoms with

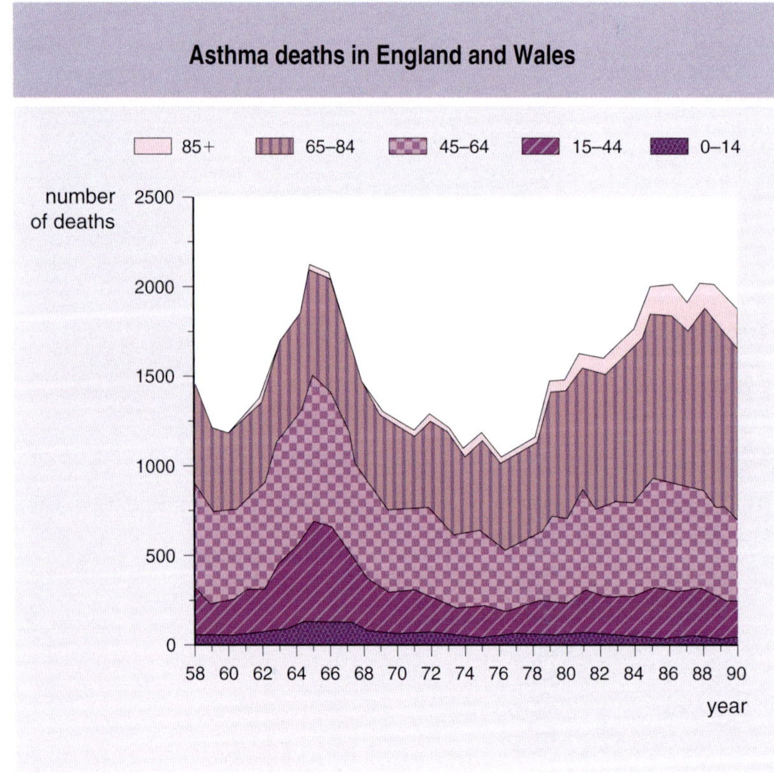

Fig. 4.1 Asthma deaths in England and Wales from 1958 to 1990, classed by age, males and females combined. (Source: OPCS.)

plugs'. If the plugs are not coughed up, the airway is blocked and the alveoli distal to the plug cease to function. In patients who have died of acute severe asthma, mucous plugging is one of the most typical features (**Figs 4.4 & 4.5**). Thus, nebulized treatments may help not only by producing bronchodilatation, but also by humidifying the airways and helping to clear the plugs.

initial assessment

Initial assessment of asthma consists of (i) checking for signs of very severe asthma (**Fig. 4.6**), (ii) measuring the PEF, and (iii) planning treatment.

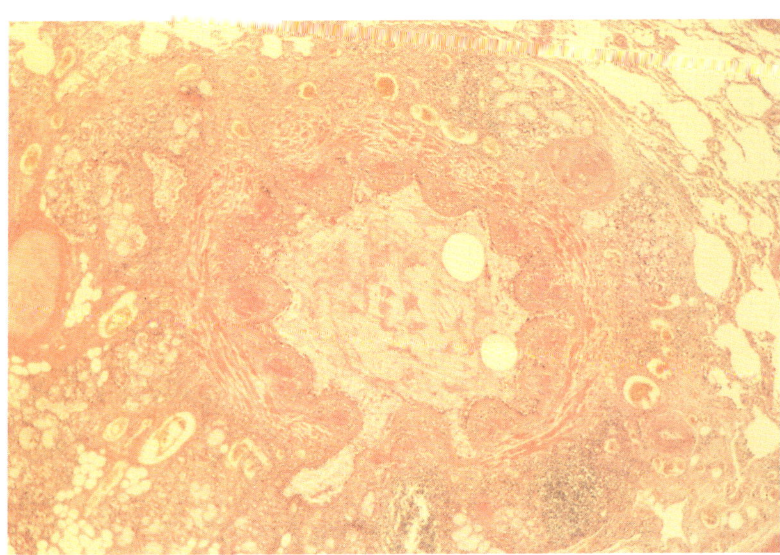

Fig. 4.5 Microscopic view of mucous plugging of the airways in acute severe asthma. Note also the epithelial disruption, basement membrane thickening and widespread infiltration with inflammatory cells.

Signs of severe asthma		
	Adults	**Children**
Severe asthma	Too wheezy or breathless to complete sentences in one breath Respiratory rate ≥ 25 breaths/min Heart rate ≥ 110 beats/min PEF ≤ 50% of predicted or best	Too breathless to talk Too breathless to feed Respiratory rate ≥ 50 breaths/min Heart rate ≥ 140 beats/min PEF ≤ 50% of best
Life–threatening attack	PEF < 33% of predicted normal or best Cyanosis, a silent chest, or feeble respiratory effort Bradycardia or hypotension Exhaustion, confusion, or syncope	PEF < 33% of best Cyanosis, a silent chest, or feeble respiratory effort Fatigue or exhaustion Agitation or reduce level of consciousness

Fig. 4.6 Signs of severe asthma.

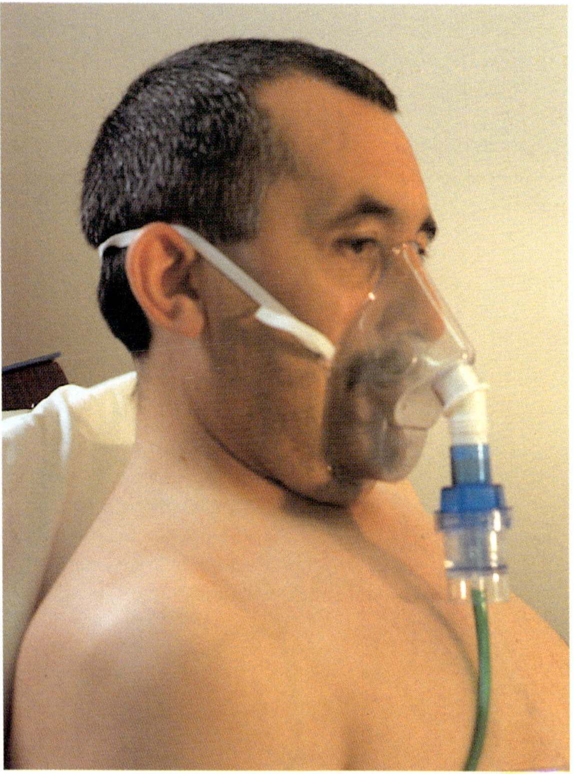

Fig. 4.7 Oxygen should be given as soon as possible to patients with acute severe asthma. The risk of significant carbon dioxide retention is very low in known asthmatics, so oxygen should be given in the highest available concentration. If it is given via a nebulizer chamber, bronchodilator therapy can be administered simultaneously.

In the most severe cases, coma or extreme distress may make PEF measurement impossible and the doctor should consider the need for intubation and emergency resuscitation (see below).

If the patient is not *in extremis*, the first therapy to be given is oxygen by mask, using the highest concentration available (**Fig. 4.7**). This should be administered without delay, either in the ambulance or on arrival in the casualty department at the hospital, while the PEF meter is being prepared for use.

objective assessment of the problem

Obtain a PEF value

Clinical signs, such as intercostal indrawing, the use of accessory muscles, an apparently hyperinflated chest, and auscultatory wheeze, may help the clinician suspect the diagnosis, but are too variable to be good indicators of severity. PEF should therefore always be measured, to confirm the nature of the problem and to provide a baseline against which to measure subsequent response to treatment (**Fig. 4.8**). It is almost always possible to measure the PEF, and pretreatment values are very useful in confirming the severity of the episode. The oxygen can be removed for a few seconds while the patient records his/her peak flow.

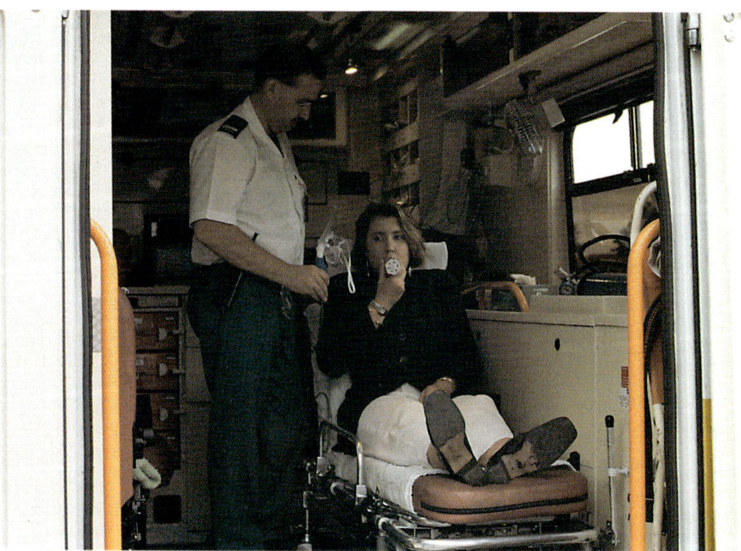

Fig. 4.8 A baseline reading of peak expiratory flow should be obtained before treatment in acute severe asthma, unless the patient is unable to co-operate. The baseline reading can be compared with subsequent readings to monitor the patient's progress.

Nebulized bronchodilator

The next stage is to give a nebulized bronchodilator. The nebulizer produces a fine mist of respirable particles containing the active drug (**Fig. 4.9**) that enables a high dose of bronchodilator to be administered quickly and effectively. In asthma, it is usual to power the nebulizer with compressed oxygen, so that the patient's oxygen requirements are met at the same time. The doses of beta-2-agonist or anticholinergic given by a nebulizer are much greater than are available from a simple pressurized metered dose inhaler (pMDI), and plasma levels of the drug are, therefore, high on the dose–response curve. A similar high dose can also be obtained by taking multiple puffs of beta -2- agonist from a pMDI connected to a large-volume spacer. Even young children can use these devices (**Fig. 4.10**). If bronchospasm is so severe that the inhaled drugs are not reaching the airways, intravenous administration of beta-2-agonists is also possible, although rarely necessary.

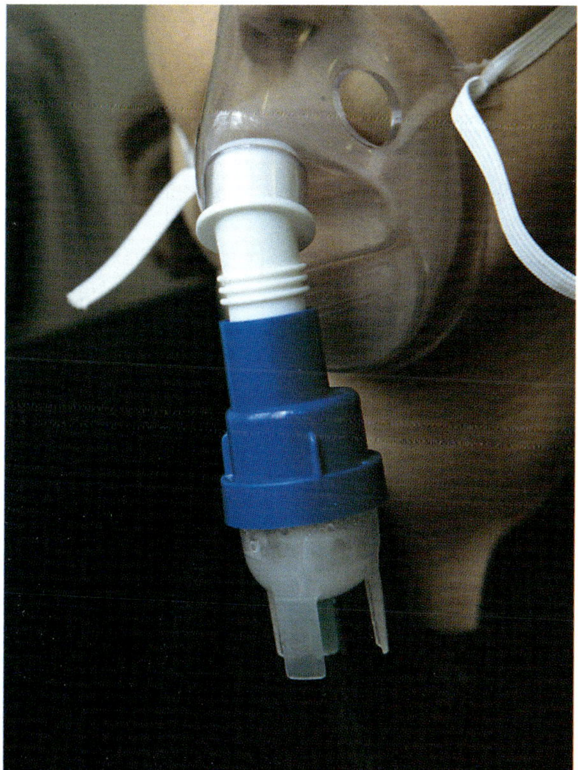

Fig. 4.9 Nebulized bronchodilator therapy is the usual immediate drug treatment for acute severe asthma. The nebulizer produces a fine mist of respirable particles containing active drug, allowing the administration of a high dose of bronchodilator quickly and without active patient co-operation.

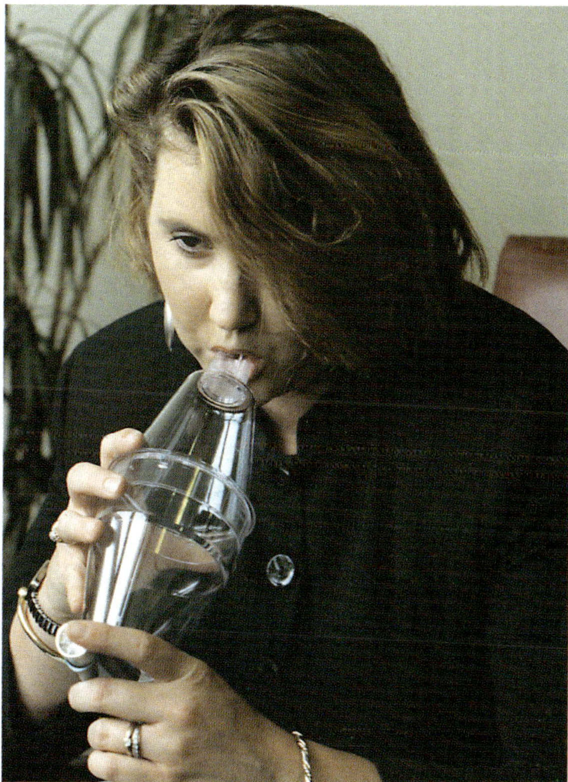

Fig. 4.10 A pMDI with a large volume spacer is an alternative method of administration of bronchodilator therapy to co-operative patients with acute severe asthma.

Systemic steroids

As for most allergic conditions, systemic steroids are highly effective and should be given immediately (**Fig. 4.11**). Even when injected, steroids do not begin to act at a cellular level for some hours, so unless there is a problem with swallowing, or potential poor absorption, they can be given orally (30–40mg of non-enteric coated prednisolone in adults and 1–2 mg/kg in children).

Secondary assessments

Measurement of oxygen saturation with a finger or ear probe is helpful (**Fig. 4.12**), whatever the level of inspired oxygen. If the saturation is greater than 92% there is no need to go on to the much more uncomfortable measurement of arterial blood gases. If oxygen saturation is <92%, arterial puncture should be done (**Fig. 4.13**) because a normal or raised pCO_2 (>5kPa) or a low pH (< 7.26) suggests significant hypoventilation, which is often a sign that the patient is tiring and thus is more likely to need intermittent positive pressure ventilation (IPPV).

While carrying out the steps above, the doctor should also be alert to other possible explanations for the patient's deterioration. Pneumothorax, which occurs in 0.5–1% of acute severe asthma admissions, is an important, treatable example (**Fig. 4.14**).

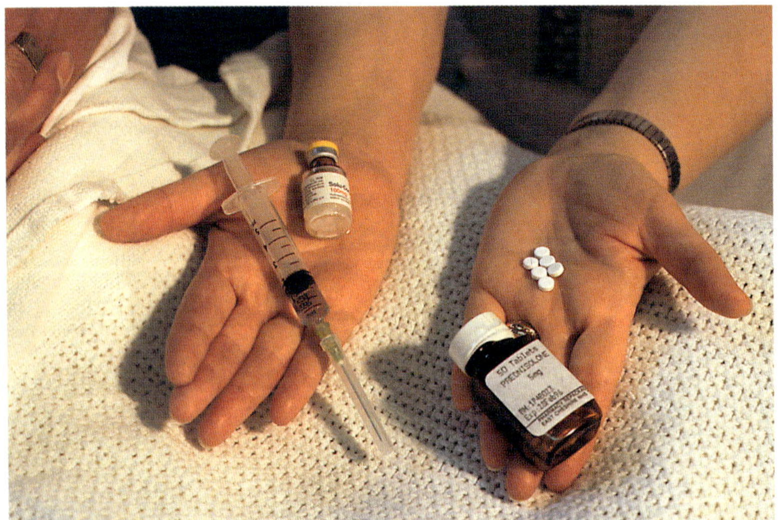

Fig. 4.11 Systemic steroid therapy should be given early in acute severe asthma. Although intravenous steroid therapy has traditionally been given, oral steroids may be just as effective in many patients.

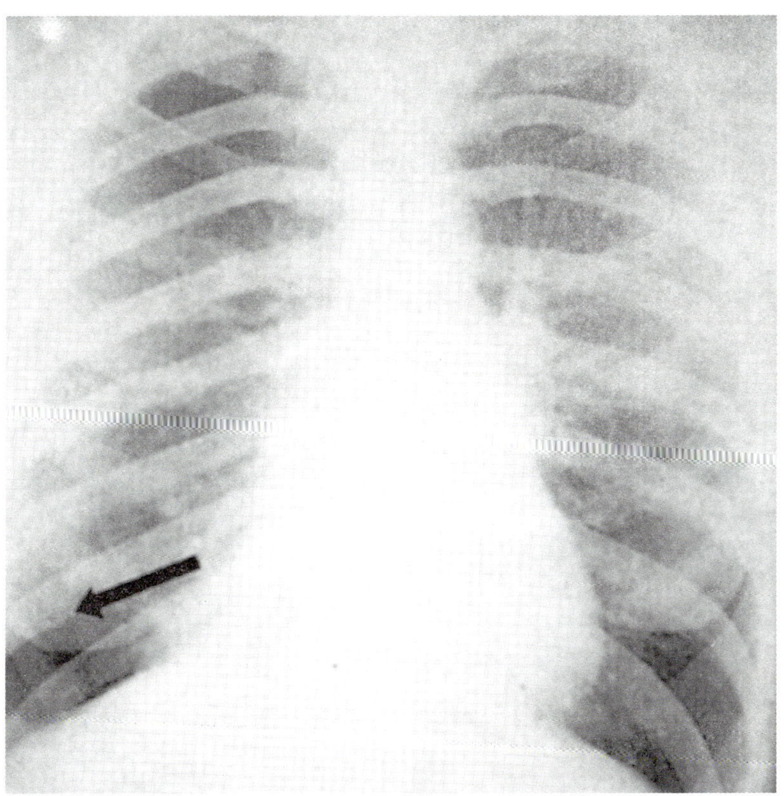

Fig. 4.12 Right sided pneumothorax in a patient with asthma. The edge of the lung is marked with an arrow. It is important to consider the possibility of other contributory factors in patients presenting with apparent acute severe asthma.

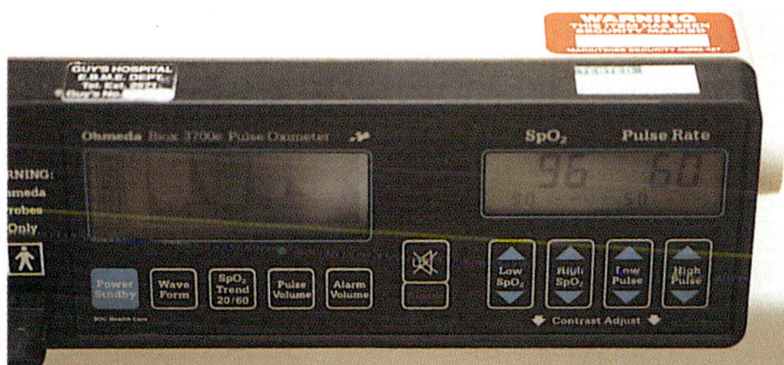

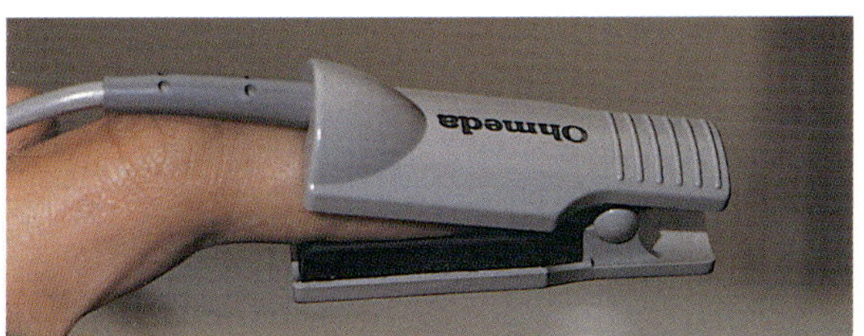

Fig. 4.13 The pulse oximeter is a valuable non-invasive method of monitoring oxygen saturation in patients with acute severe asthma. The device is accurate at the levels of oxygen saturation seen in most patients with asthma (over 80% saturation) if cardiac output and local circulation are adequate. If the measured saturation is 92% or below, however, this should be confirmed by arterial puncture.

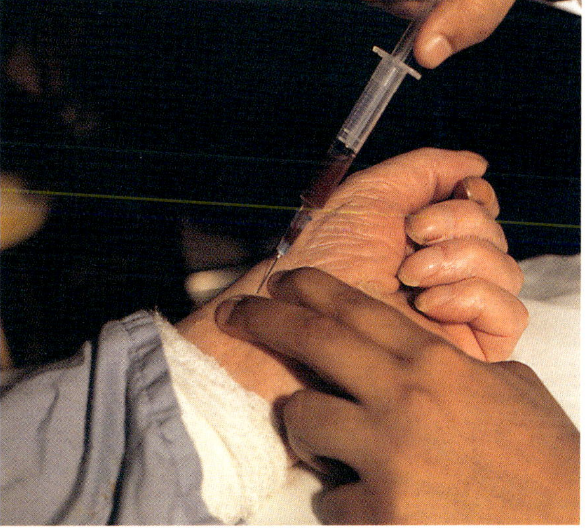

Fig. 4.14 Arterial blood gas estimation is indicated in patients with severe acute asthma whose oxygen saturation is 92% or below, and in confused or drowsy patients.

initiate treatment based on PEF (% predicted)

The PEF should be repeated 10–15 minutes after the first use of the nebulizer (**Fig. 4.15**). If levels are no better then the nebulized beta-2-agonist can be repeated and an anticholinergic added, mixed in the same nebulizer (**Fig. 4.16**).

If the patient is still not improving and has not developed any of the signs of life-threatening asthma, then there are a number of therapeutic options to consider. These include using continuously nebulized salbutamol in a lower dose (diluted 1:50) via an ultrasonic nebulizer, or giving aminophylline intravenously in a dose of 0.5 μg/kg/min in a continuous infusion (**Fig. 4.17**) Arterial blood gases should be checked if there no improvement in PEF, or if the initial PEF values were abnormal.

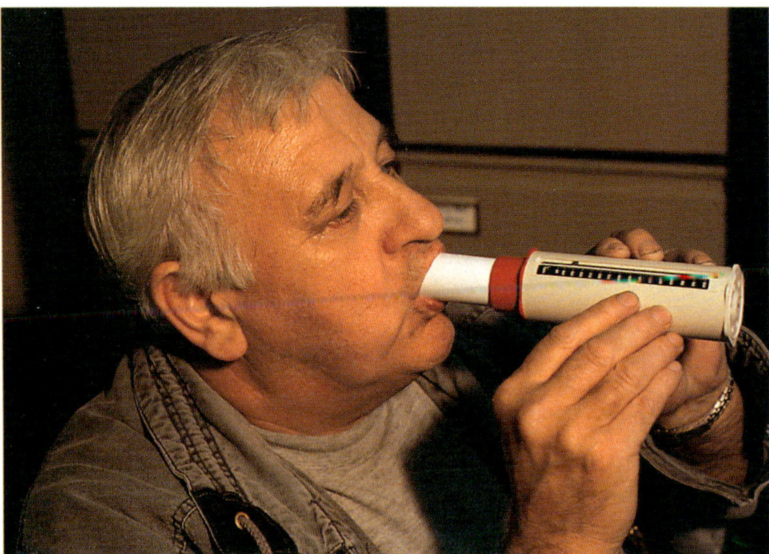

Fig. 4.15 The PEF should be repeated in acute severe asthma after initial treatment with a nebulized bronchodilator. If the PEF remains low, further bronchodilator treatment is indicated.

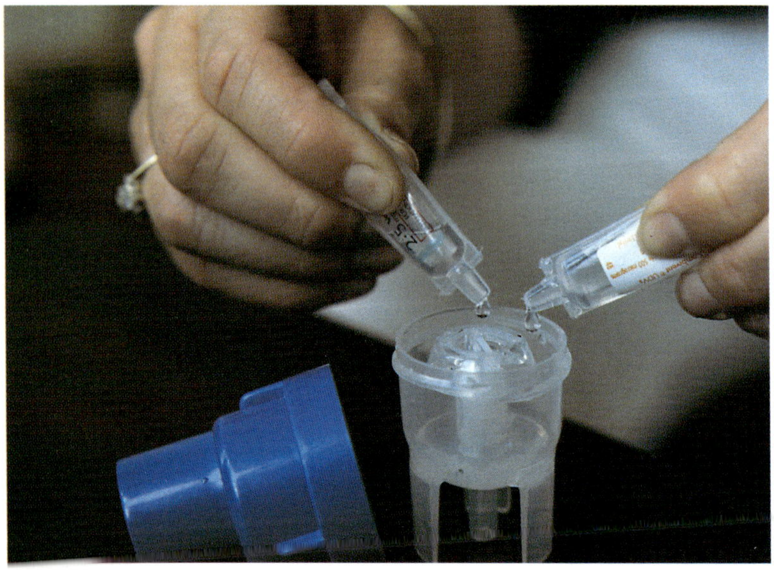

Fig. 4.16 Chemically compatible drugs can be mixed in the nebulizer chamber. Here salbutamol (a beta-2-agonist) and ipratropium bromide (an anticholinergic) are being mixed for simultaneous administration.

initiate treatment based on PEF (% predicted)

The above measures will stabilize most asthma episodes, and progressive improvement over the next 24–48 hours is usual. Continued therapy consists of oxygen as long as the arterial oxygen saturation on air is low, 4–6 hourly nebulized bronchodilators, and oral prednisolone. Inhaled steroids should be commenced or recommenced as soon as the patient is physically able to use an ordinary inhaler. The dose should be higher than the patient's previous dose. Patients improving in this way can be discharged.

Patients with post-treatment PEF values less than 50% of predicted are treated with nebulized bronchodilators and systemic steroids, and kept in the hospital.

A patient deteriorating at any time in spite of treatment should be managed as for a very severe attack.

For the patient arriving in hospital with signs of life-threatening asthma, or who deteriorates in spite of therapy, the approach is rather different.

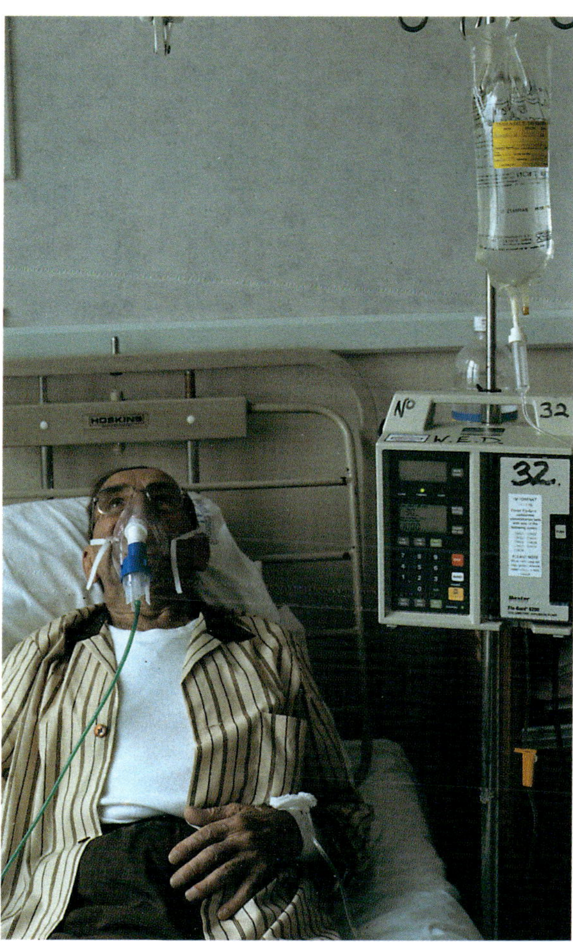

Fig. 4.17 Intravenous aminophylline may be administered by slow intravenous infusion in patients who respond poorly to initial treatment with a beta-2-agonist. The dose must be carefully checked, and serum theophylline levels should be estimated, if this form of therapy is continued for 24 hours or more.

The patient who is comatose or has failing consciousness needs to be treated with IPPV without delay (**Figs 4.18 & 4.19**) In less critically ill patients the need for IPPV is largely dictated by the arterial blood gas measurements. Carbon dioxide retention ($PaCO_2$ > 6kPa) or acidosis (pH < 7.26) suggest that the patient is tiring and that there is an imminent risk of complete respiratory failure. Unless there is a dramatic response to nebulizers, oxygen and steroids, IPPV will be necessary.

patient admitted to hospital

Most asthma attacks subside over 24–48 hours. The improvement can be monitored with a four-hourly peak flow chart recorded before and after the nebulized bronchodilators (**Fig. 4.20**). It is helpful to mark on the chart the patient's previous best PEF value (or if this is not known,

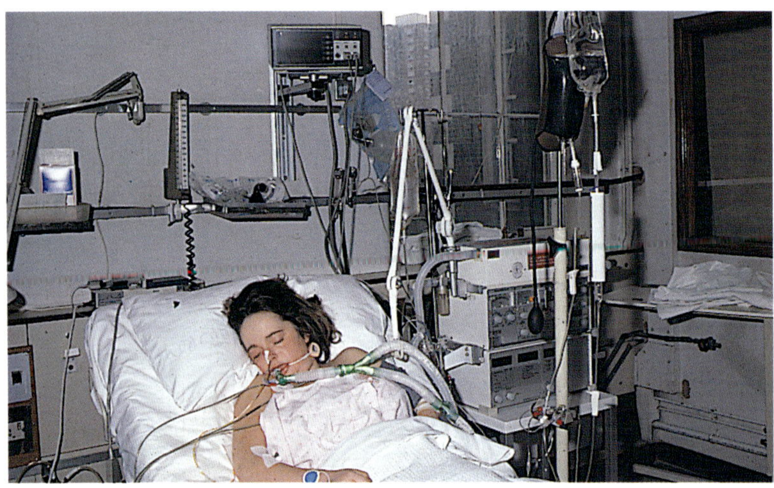

Fig. 4.18 Ventilation of a patient with severe acute asthma. Intermittent positive pressure ventilation is indicated when respiratory exhaustion occurs, with a falling PaO_2 in the presence of a rising $PaCO_2$ or acidosis (pH < 7.26). Supportive ventilation may correct these abnormalities, and allows bronchodilators and steroids time to take effect.

Indications for intensive care
Deteriorating peak flow, worsening or persisting hypoxia (PaO_2 < 8kPa) despite 60% inspired oxygen, or hypercapnia ($PaCO_2$ > 6kPa)
Onset of exhaustion, feeble respiration, confusion, or drowsiness
Coma or respiratory arrest
Indications for intermittent positive pressure ventilation (IPPV)
A proportion of patients with the above indications will not respond quickly in the ITU. Non-response strongly indicates the need for intubation. Asthma patients are not easy to intubate and ventilate and the procedure should be performed by an anaesthetist

Fig. 4.19 Indications for intensive care.

the predicted value) so that there is a clear target relevant to that patient. The following treatment plan is for a typical adult asthmatic who will be ready for discharge at 4–5 days. As the patient improves, the extra therapy can be progressively withdrawn.

If the PEF values are clearly improving at 24 hours then the nebulized anticholinergic can be withdrawn. As the PEF values approach the patient's best recorded value, the nebulized beta-agonist can be exchanged for an ordinary inhaler. This is an opportunity to re-evaluate the patient's ability to use the inhaler.

About half of all asthmatics fail to use a pMDI correctly. It is unwise to assume that because a person has had an inhaler for some time, they will necessarily be

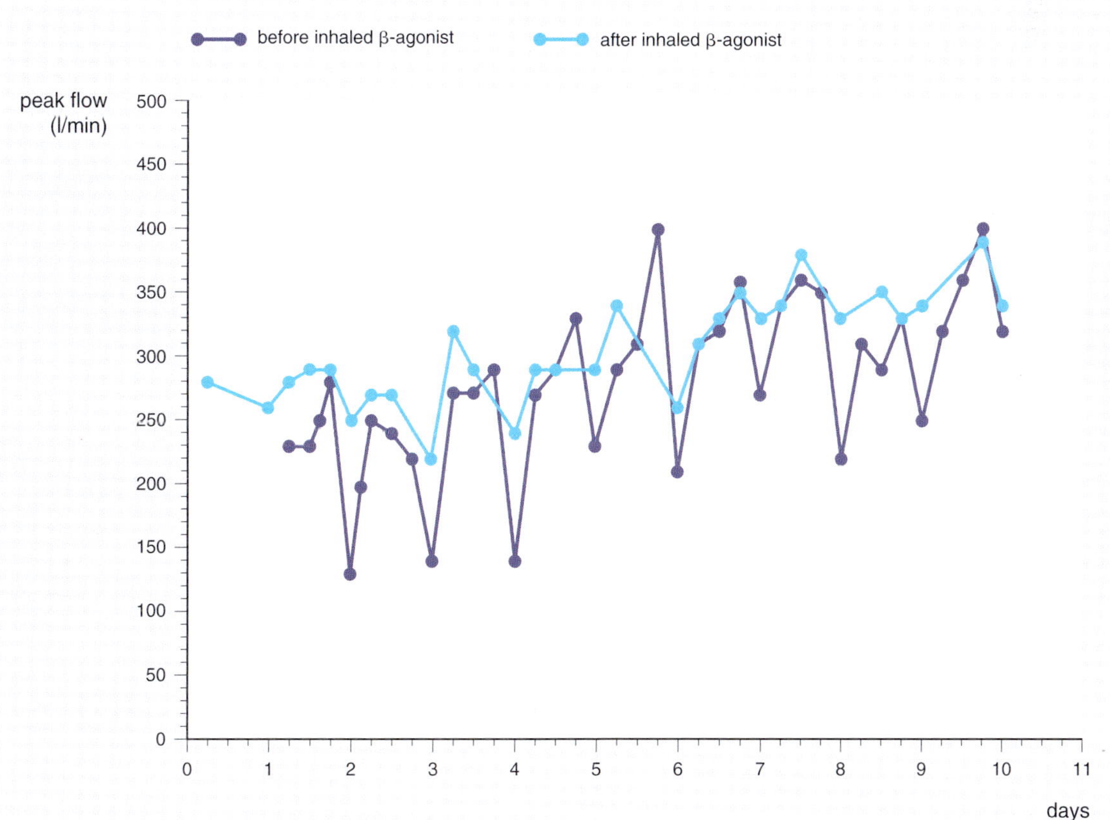

Fig. 4.20 Recovery from acute severe asthma may be monitored by regular recordings of PEF. PEF should be measured before and after the administration of nebulized bronchodilator therapy, and monitoring continued throughout the patient's stay in hospital. This patient's previous best PEF was 425 L/min.

competent in its use. Inhaler technique is often overlooked, but should be part of every doctor's routine when reassessing the asthmatic's progress. Some asthma units make it part of the nurse's responsibility when giving out medication to also check on inhaler technique, just as they would check that patients had actually swallowed any tablets prescribed.

assessment for discharge

Asthma is a chronic disorder, and is not cured by acute admission to hospital. Assessment for discharge therefore aims to ensure not only that the acute episode has been successfully treated, but also that future morbidity is prevented. A series of questions should be asked of the patient prior to discharge from hospital (**Fig. 4.21**).

Has this attack settled?

Assessment of fitness may appear relatively easy in younger subjects, for whom the transformation between admission and discharge is very marked. However, daytime assessments may overlook important diurnal variations unless the PEF chart is examined. Peak flow variability (**Fig. 4.22**) is a useful objective measure of the underlying asthma volatility. If the PEF variability is high, this suggests a greater degree of underlying lability of

Pre-discharge assessment	
Has acute episode settled?	Symptoms of wheeze and breathlessness settled Slept well on preceding night PEF chart shows values at or close to the individual's known best (or predicted value if the best value not known) PEF chart does not show excessive PEF variability
Was there an identifiable cause for this episode?	Exposure to an asthmogen at work Is there a cat or dog at home? Are reasonable dust mite reduction measures possible in the home? Has the person been suffering from a cold or other viral infection?
Was treatment optimum before this episode?	Had the patient run out of inhalers and if so was the problem (i) due to the patient's forgetfulness or (ii) due to inadequate access to the clinic that provides the prescription? Had the patient been prescribed a steroid inhaler, and were they using it? Did the patient have access to oral steroids in the few days that the attack was developing?
Did the patient know how to recognize the acute attack developing?	Did the patient record their PEF as symptoms began? Is the patient aware of the significance of particular reductions in PEF? Did the patient react appropriately to the falling PEF?
Did the patient's relatives or carers know how to recognize and react to the acute episode?	This is particularly important in cases of acute brittle asthma

Fig. 4.21 Pre-discharge assessment following admission for acute severe asthma.

the airways. It has been shown that patients with PEF variability greater than 20–25% are more likely to be readmitted with a further episode in the next few months. Guidelines suggest that patients with PEF variability greater than 25% should only be discharged after formal reassessment, and should be provided with a clear management plan. Although most patients are stable by 5 days, some take much longer (**Fig. 4.23**).

Is the patient established on the right therapy?

The patient should have been moved from nebulizer onto ordinary inhalers, used as required, at least 24 hours and usually 48 hours before discharge. This is to ensure that

PEF variability

PEF variability is calculated from the PEF measurements made in the previous 24 hours and is defined in the British asthma guidelines as:

$$\text{PEF variability} = \left(\frac{\text{best PEF} - \text{lowest PEF}}{\text{best PEF}}\right) \times 100$$

Values above 25% are said to be abnormal. Since the measurement is based only on 24 hours data, the clinician needs to interpret the results in the light of the rest of the clinical picture

Fig. 4.22 PEF variability is a useful objective measure of the underlying volatility of asthma.

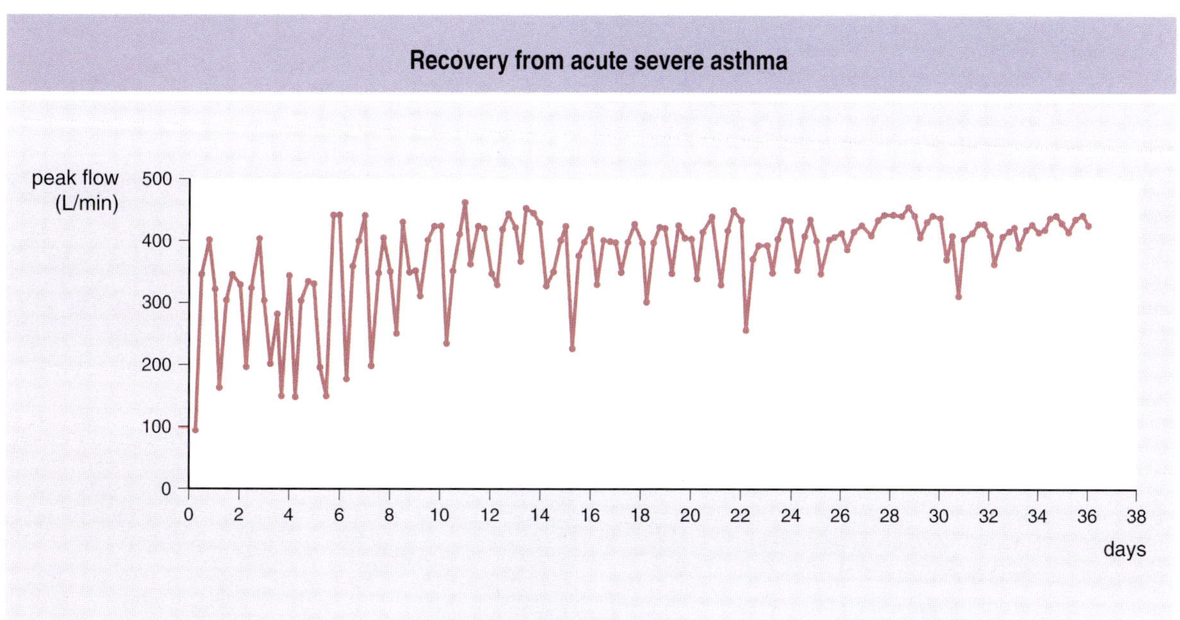

Fig. 4.23 PEF variability following an attack of acute severe asthma may take some time to return to pre-attack levels.

the reduction in dose is not associated with a serious deterioration in function, and allows the clinician to check that the patient is able to use the inhaler correctly. Despite tuition, many patients have difficulty using pMDIs; if this is observed on the ward then the device can be changed to one that the patient can use (**Fig. 4.24**).

There is a bewildering range of different inhalers and attachments available (*see* Chapter 2). The doctor or nurse should ensure that the patient is competent using the prescribed device. If the patient is not happy with the device, an alternative should be sought. Pressurized metered dose inhalers are the cheapest, but are also the most difficult to use correctly. Breath-actuated pMDIs are easier to use and are less likely to be incorrectly used. Dry powder inhalers (DPIs) are increasingly used, and are most likely to be used correctly. However, it is not appropriate to give everyone these more expensive devices since, with good teaching, many patients master the pMDI, especially when used in conjunction with a large volume spacer. Children as young as four years old can often use these spacer devices (**Fig. 4.25**).

All patients should be on some sort of asthma prophylaxis following an attack requiring hospitalization. Guidelines recommend that the patient is kept on oral steroids for up to three weeks (**Fig. 4.26**). This helps to ensure that airway inflammation has time to resolve, and it is also important that patients go home on a dose of inhaled steroid that is higher than their pre-admission dose.

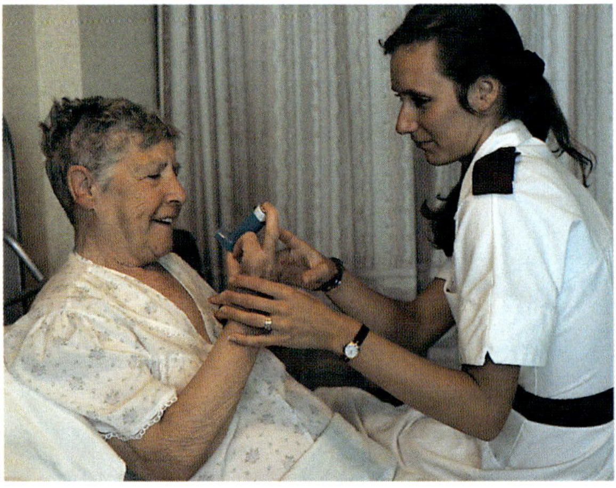

Fig. 4.24 Teaching and monitoring of inhaler technique is an essential part of the preparation of the patient for discharge from hospital.

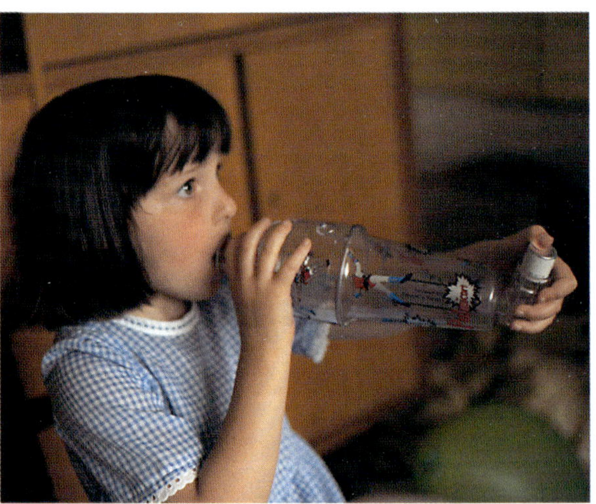

Fig. 4.25 A large volume spacer device attached to a pMDI is a particularly good method of delivering therapy to young children.

Was the patient's previous therapy adequate?

The dose of prophylactic therapy should be higher than that taken prior to admission. There are important additional questions to ask about the patient's compliance. Many patients claim to take their prophylactic inhalers regularly; studies have shown that the truth is often very different. One way of checking compliance is to check the collection of prescriptions, which can often be done from computerized prescribing records.

A patient who was non-compliant with therapy prior to their attack should be followed up with great care. Reasons for non-compliance are poorly understood and range from simple forgetfulness to a fear of side-effects of inhaled steroids. Patients' worries, fears and understanding need to be carefully and systematically explored and, if possible, answered.

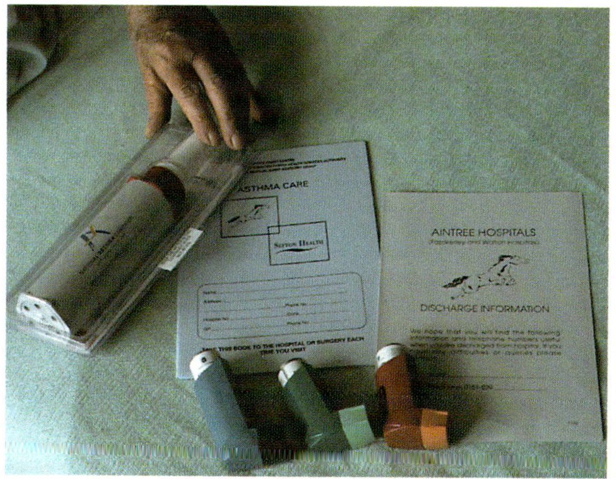

Fig. 4.26 Typical therapy on discharge of a patient with acute severe asthma from hospital. The oral steroid therapy will be gradually withdrawn, while control is maintained by inhaled steroid therapy (brown inhaler) and occasional relief therapy is provided by an inhaled beta-2-agonist (blue inhaler).

Recognition of worsening asthma – designing a self management plan

An asthmatic may feel unwell for many reasons, many of which are unconnected with the asthma. The only sure way of knowing if asthma is getting out of control is self-measurement of peak flow. If peak flows are recorded during a period of good health then the patient's best PEF value can be determined. When values fall below this value, the asthma is probably deteriorating. This simple approach can create a self-management plan for the patient to follow, so that he/she takes charge of his/her condition for much of the time. A typical self-management plan links a series of peak flow values calculated from the patient's best known value, to specific actions designed to abort the acute attack (**Fig. 4.27**). However, the plan also makes it clear that if the patient is not responding, or if the PEF is less than 50% of the patient's best value

Self-management plan

Your doctor or nurse will complete this page with you

SELF-MANAGEMENT PLAN

personal best peak flow . . . .

When you feel well and your peak flow is . . . . (above 80%)	Continue your usual treatment . . . .
When your asthma starts to get worse, e.g. • it wakes you at night • you need more reliever treatment • you get cold *or* • your peak flow drops below . . . . (80%)	Add/increase your preventer treatment . . . . until you are completely better. Then go back to usual treatment
If you don't improve or continue to feel worse *or* your peak flow drops below . . . . (60%)	Continue above treatment and take a short course of oral steroids (prednisolone) i.e. . . . . tablets every day before breakfast until you are completely better. Contact your nurse/doctor for a check up
If you are distressed and/or your inhaler gives no relief or peak flow drops to . . . . (50%)	Contact your doctor urgently, or go to hospital (accident and emergency department)

This is a severe attack – dial 999

This management plan must be reviewed yearly

Fig. 4.27 A self-management plan should be developed by the patient with a specialized asthma nurse and/or a physician. Each plan should be unique to the patient.

Precipitating factors in anaphylactic reactions	
Factor	**Examples**
Drugs	Aspirin, NSAIDs, anaesthetics, antibiotics, induction agents and muscle relaxants
Diagnostic agents	Radio-opaque dyes
Vitamins	Folic acid, thiamine
Hormones	ACTH, insulin, methylprednisolone, parathormone, oestradiol
Enzymes	Asparaginase, chymopapain, chymotrypsin, penicillinase, trypsin
Allergen extracts	Epidermal extracts, house dust mite, pollens
Horse antiserum	Antilymphocytic globulin, venom antitoxin
Blood products	Blood, cryoprecipitate, immunoglobulin
Venoms	Bee and wasp venom
Foods	Peanut, egg, milk, nuts, shellfish, soy bean
Miscellaneous	Dextran, seminal fluid, latex

Fig. 5.1 Precipitating factors in anaphylactic reactions.

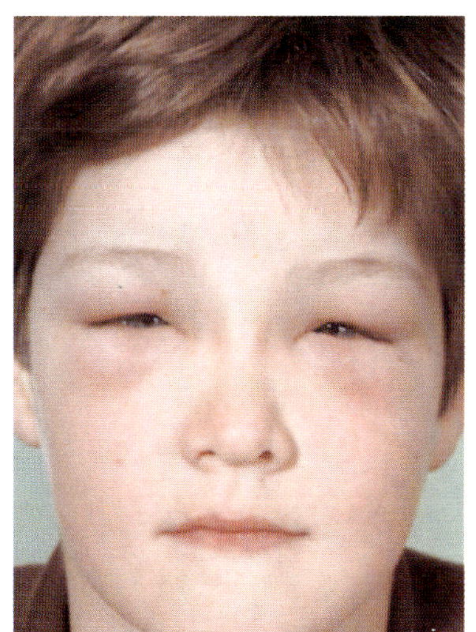
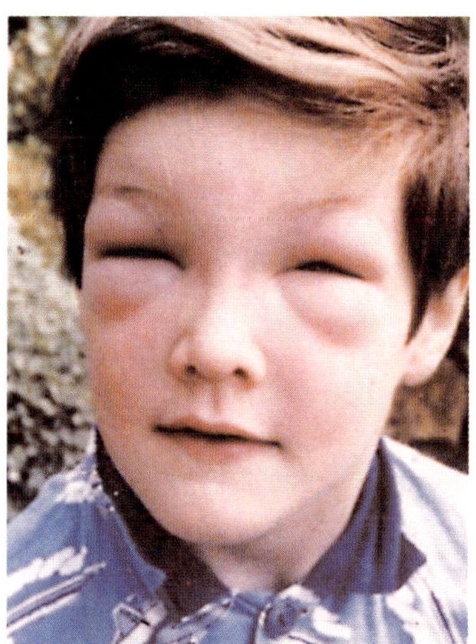
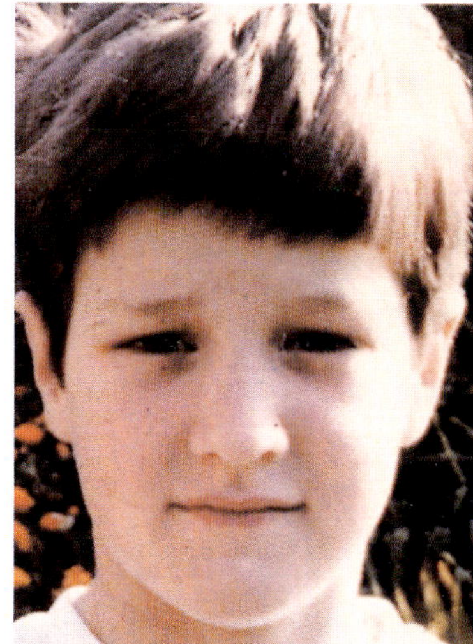

Fig. 5.2 Severe angioedema in a nine-year-old boy following a bee sting. This child had been stung several times in early childhood without developing a systemic reaction. Left: Two hours after a bee sting he suffered severe angioedema of the face, but no systemic reaction. Centre: Some weeks later he was stung again and developed a more severe angioedema, which developed into an anaphylactic reaction with larygeal oedema and bronchospasm. Right: Normal appearance following recovery. Note that the appearance of angioedema (left) does not mean that subsequent reactions will necessarily be more severe, but it is a risk factor.

5 Anaphylactic Reactions

Lawrence Youlten

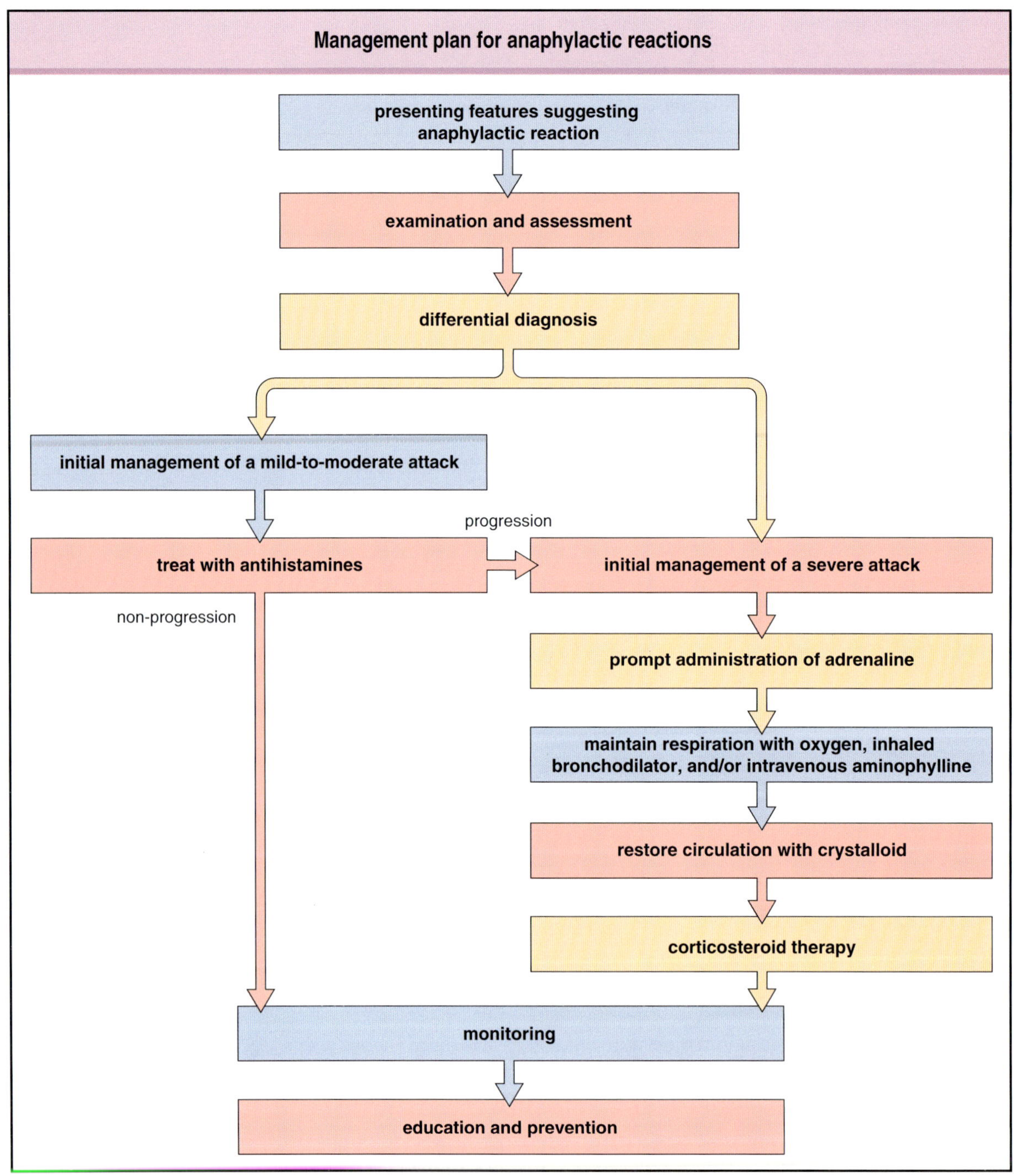

An anaphylactic reaction may be preceded by prodromal symptoms (**Fig. 5.3**). These symptoms include many classic symptoms of allergic reactions: pruritus, urticaria, rhinitis, conjunctivitis, periorbital oedema, and excess production of tears. If the reaction is very mild, it may not proceed to a full blown attack, and recedes after a few minutes or hours. It is important at this stage to determine the cause of the reaction, as a subsequent attack may be more serious.

Mild or prodomal symptoms of an anaphylactic reaction
Light-headedness
Warmth, tingling, itch, weals
Feeling of 'dullness' in the ears
'Pins and needles', often around the mouth
Eye irritation and swelling
Nasal symptoms (itchy nose, blocked nose, hypersecretion, sneezing)

Fig. 5.3 Mild or prodromal symptoms of an anaphylactic reaction.

Systemic effects of a full-blown anaphylactic reaction

System	Clinical features
Skin and mucous membranes	Generalized flushing, itching and swelling
Respiratory tract	Oedema of mouth, pharynx and larynx, hoarseness, stridor/wheezing, bronchospasm, respiratory arrest
Cardiovascular system	Myocardial ischaemia, arrhythmias, cardiac arrest, hypotension
Gastrointestinal tract	Nausea, vomiting, tenesmus, diarrhoea
Genitourinary system	Uterine cramps, urinary incontinence
Nervous system	Anxiety, convulsions

Fig. 5.4 Systemic effects of a full-blown anaphylactic reaction.

5 Anaphylactic Reactions

Lawrence Youlten

Introduction

An anaphylactic reaction in immunological terms is the mechanism by which a Type I ('immediate') hypersensitivity reaction causes generalized IgE-mediated inflammation following absorption of an allergen. When the effects are confined to a weal and flare reaction at the contact site, the term 'local anaphylactic reaction' is sometimes used.

As a clinical term, 'anaphylactic reaction' describes a pattern of symptomatology which may include bronchial constriction, laryngeal oedema, hypotension, urticaria, and angioedema. These symptoms are often severe and sometimes fatal, and require immediate treatment if the survival of the patient is to be assured.

The true prevalence of anaphylaxis is unknown, as it seems likely that many mild-to-moderate reactions go unreported. The more reliable data relate principally to fatalities. Penicillin injections are the leading cause of mortality and morbidity, with 10–40 cases per 100 000 injections, and 100–500 deaths per year in the USA. Stings from hymenoptera cause approximately 40 deaths per year in the USA, while the risk of non-fatal anaphylaxis following stings is estimated at less than 1%.

Because anaphylactic reactions are rare, few people can be said to be experienced in their treatment. It is estimated that the average general practitioner (GP) in Britain can expect to see one case every 56 years. However, since this one case may be precipitated by the doctor, for example following an immunization injection, and because it may well be a life-threatening situation, it is important that the management of anaphylactic reactions is understood.

presenting features suggesting anaphylactic reaction

Likely precipitating factors

A list of potential precipitating factors is given in **Fig. 5.1** The allergens most likely to be administered by medical personnel are small-to-medium sized proteins (e.g. hormones, vaccines, enzymes, and blood products), but a variety of non-protein drugs (e.g. penicillin and other antibiotics, aspirin) can also precipitate the reaction.

Common environmental factors include hymenoptera stings (usually from bees or wasps; **Fig. 5.2**), and certain food products, in particular peanuts and egg white. Exercise, sometimes in conjunction with particular food allergies, may be a precipitant. Recently, latex has been increasingly recognised as an allergen which can produce systemic as well as local anaphylactic reactions. Surgical gloves, the powder from them, and condoms have all been associated with anaphylactic reactions.

A history of atopy confers a minimal additional risk of an attack, but may be associated with increased severity of reactions when they occur. There appear to be no other significant predisposing factors. Factors having no proven correlation with the incidence or risk of anaphylactic reaction include age, race, occupation, and time of year. Mastocytosis may present as repeated anaphylactic episodes triggered by allergic, toxic, chemical or physical triggers.

Clinical features

The time of onset of anaphylactic reactions varies, and is a guide to the severity of the reaction that will follow. Thus, systemic symptoms occurring within 10 minutes of exposure indicate a very serious reaction, requiring prompt and appropriate therapy. Less severe attacks can take up to 60 minutes to develop. Reactions to food or to slow release tablets may take even longer.

The symptoms of a full blown anaphylactic reaction can involve many organ systems (**Fig. 5.4**). Urticaria is a common feature (**Fig. 5.5**), and is sometimes accompanied by angioedema (**Fig. 5.6**). Angioedema in the mouth, tongue, pharynx or throat can endanger the patency of the upper airways. If untreated, this leads to hoarseness, stridor, and cyanosis, and is potentially fatal. Involvement of the lower airways is evidenced by dyspnoea, tightness of the chest, and bronchospasm. Cardiovascular symptoms (arrhythmias, myocardial ischaemia, hypotension) can occur very rapidly, and may be the only signs of an anaphylactic reaction. Although the majority of cases will demonstrate several of these symptoms, and sometimes also symptoms in the gastrointestinal tract and the genitourinary and nervous systems, occasional patients will show evidence only of shock.

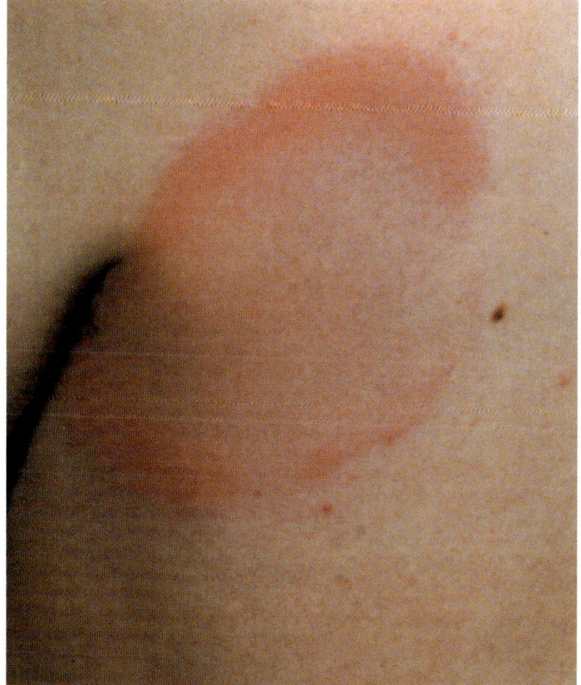

Fig. 5.5 Urticaria is a common presentation of sensitivity to penicillin. This case was associated with amoxycillin in a 24-year-old man.

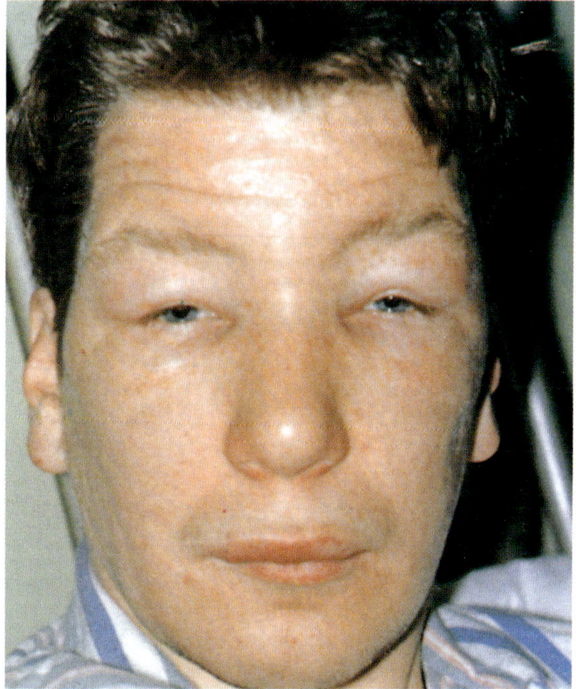

Fig. 5.6 Angioedema following penicillin ingestion is not uncommon. It may be associated with laryngeal oedema or anaphylaxis and should be treated promptly.

Although the onset of clinical findings is usually abrupt, they may be delayed when, for example, the reaction follows absorption of an orally administered antigen. Significant delayed mortality and morbidity may also occur, owing to impaired perfusion of vital organs during the acute phase of anaphylactic shock. Biphasic anaphylactic reactions, analagous to late-phase reactions in other forms of Type I hypersensitivity, have also been reported. These reports have not been well verified, and the so-called second phase may sometimes represent an incomplete response to partial therapy during prolonged, severe episodes.

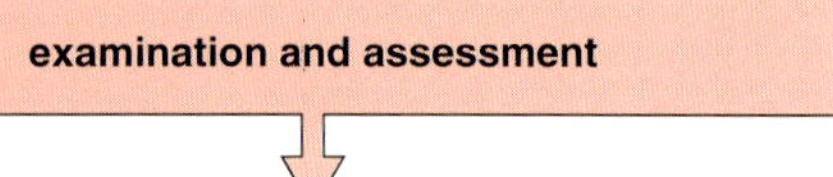

Patients with a suspected anaphylactic reaction should be briefly examined to see if they are carrying a MedicAlert bracelet (or equivalent) that might indicate what precipitated the attack.

Blood pressure, pulse rate, peak expiratory flow (PEF) and pulse oximetry (oxygen saturation) readings should be taken at the earliest possible moment, so that baseline values for the attack are established and progress can be monitored. Blood pressure will be initially low (< 100 mmHg systolic), and pulse rate will be high (>100bpm in adults). Oxygen saturation will be somewhat below the reference range of 95–98%. Subsequently, bradycardia in response to the hypoxia may be seen.

Once the patient is stable, a 10 ml clotted blood sample may be taken for the mast cell tryptase test, which is one of the few relevant laboratory investigations. This test measures levels of mast cell tryptase, a substance present in normal blood at very low concentrations, but which is seen in large concentrations in persons with a systemic anaphylactic reaction (**Fig. 5.7**). Mast cell tryptase cannot be generated as a result of handling the blood sample, and concentrations in the blood remain high for up to 6 hours after onset. However, this test has been validated only in severe reactions.

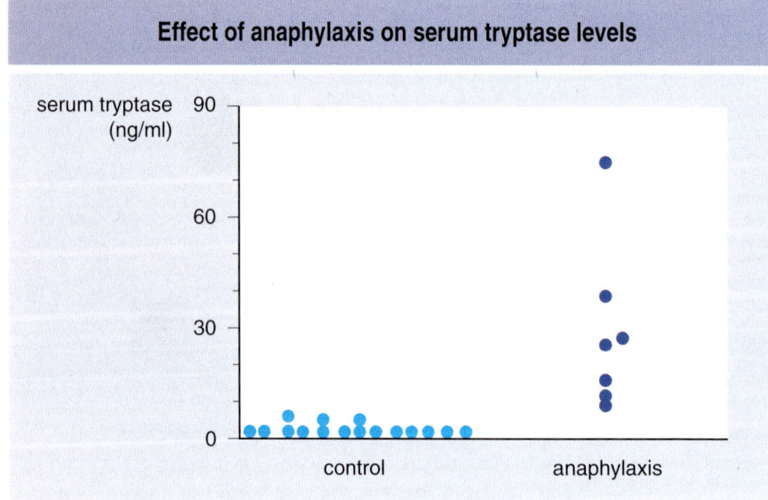

Fig. 5.7 Anaphylaxis is associated with an increase in serum tryptase levels. (Data from Schwartz *et al. N Engl J Med* 1987; **316**: 1622–1626.)

differential diagnosis

Anaphylaxis should always be considered in the differential diagnosis of a patient presenting with shock. Although the diagnosis is usually obvious – for example when the symptoms immediately follow a bee sting or a vaccination – some difficulties can arise when only one or two systems are involved, or when the patient is unconscious. Possible alternative diagnoses are listed in **Fig. 5.8**.

initial management of a mild-to-moderate attack

Where the reaction is mild or moderate in severity, the patient should be placed in the recumbent position to minimize potential complications (e.g. fainting) in the event of hypotension. Patients with airway obstruction are more comfortable propped up, but faint or unconscious patients should be prone.

Differential diagnosis

Diagnosis	Associated with	Not associated with
Vasovagal attack (usually following an injection)	Pallor, cold sweat, bradycardia, rapid recovery once prone	Severe hypotension, skin rashes or itch
Hypervontilation or other anxiety-related reactions	Fainting, hypertension, paraesthesias, a history of similar attacks	Skin rashes or itch, objective evidence of respiratory, cardiovascular or neurological problems
Myocardial infarction	Central crushing chest pain, sometimes radiating into the neck or arms	Upper airway oedema, bronchospasm, urticaria
Hypoglycaemia	Diabetes, unconsciousness preceded (sometimes) by confusion, weakness, sweating and pallor	Severe hypotension, skin rashes or itch, respiratory distress

Other potential differential diagnoses include foreign body aspiration, pulmonary embolism, acute asthma, cold urticaria, cardiac arrhythmia, cerebrovascular accident, epilepsy, hereditary angioedema, systemic mastocytosis, carcinoid syndrome, and toxic shock syndrome.

Fig. 5.8 Differential diagnosis.

Where possible, the causal agent should be removed. Bee stings remaining in the skin (**Fig. 5.9**) should be taken out carefully, so that the venom sac is not compressed to release further antigen at the site. Where the precipitating factor is suspected to be a continuously administered drug or contrast medium, administration should stop immediately.

If the site of administration is on a limb, a tourniquet can be used to slow down the rate of systemic antigen distribution. Great care must be taken to ensure that the tourniquet is loosened at regular intervals, and that ischaemic damage is prevented.

treat with antihistamines

H_1 antihistamines are effective treatments for mild reactions such as flush, itch, urticaria, and rhinitis. Chlorpheniramine is commonly used because it is injectable. Intravenous administration should be slow, i.e. over a period of 60 seconds or more. Also, because older antihistamines have a less specific H_1 activity, they have other effects that may be beneficial. However, patients receiving chlorpheniramine should be warned about possible sedative effects. Note that many antihistamines are not recommended for use in children. Physicians are personally responsible for injecting in this group.

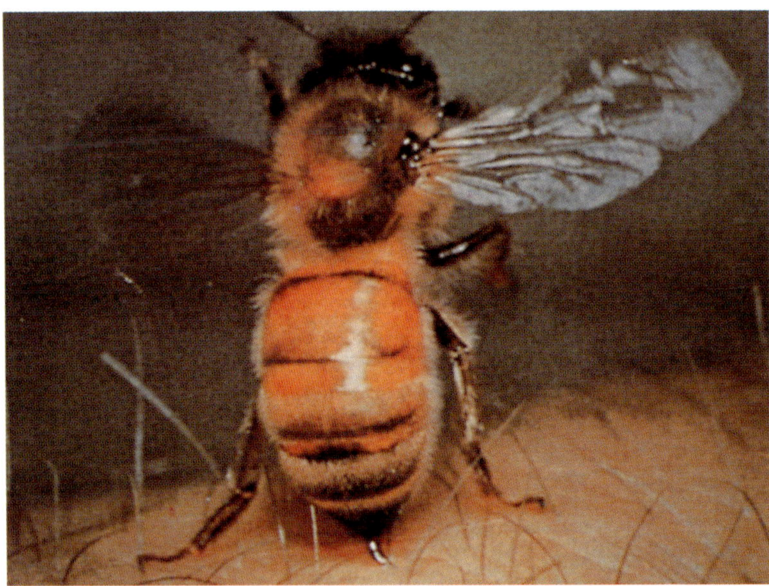

Fig. 5.9 Stings by bees and wasps are an important cause of anaphylactic reactions. When the sting is from a bee (pictured here), the sting is likely to remain in the patient and should be carefully removed. Wasp stings are not normally left behind by the insect.

initial management of a severe attack

Prompt recognition and treatment of an anaphylactic reaction can save the patient's life. However, certain risk factors increase the risk of death, particularly if the physician is unaware of their possible effects (**Fig. 5.10**).

Most mortality and morbidity in people with anaphylactic reactions is due to airway obstruction or cardiovascular collapse. Therapy, therefore, aims to preserve the patency of the airway (**Fig. 5.11**), reverse bronchospasm, and maintain blood pressure and tissue perfusion.

In a very severe, life-threatening attack, the patient may quickly lose consciousness. In such cases, resuscitative measures should begin immediately. Once the patency of the airway has been assured, and an intravenous line installed, oxygen therapy can begin. An ECG monitor allows arrhythmias to be detected and promptly treated. Adrenaline (epinephrine) and other drugs should be administered as appropriate (see below).

Risk factors for fatal anaphylactic reactions

Risk factor	Cause of death
Asthma in the young	Respiratory failure, asphyxia
Cardiovascular disease in older patients	Myocardial infarction, cerebral hypoxia
Beta-blocker therapy	General increase in the severity of the reaction

Fig. 5.10 Risk factors for fatal anaphylactic reactions.

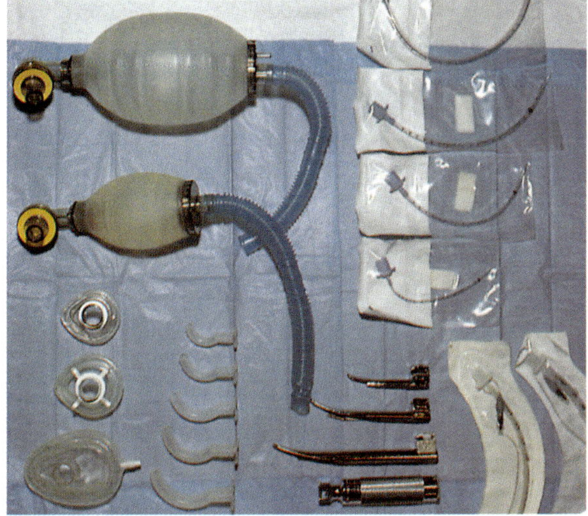

Fig. 5.11 Equipment to maintain the patency of the airway in patients with anaphylactic reaction.

prompt administration of adrenaline

Adrenaline is the mainstay of treatment in severe anaphylactic reactions. It inhibits further release of mediators from mast cells and is a powerful stimulant to the cardiovascular system, increasing cardiac output, and at the same time increasing peripheral resistance and dilating constricted airways. Prompt intramuscular or subcutaneous administration of 300–500 μg (adult dose) adrenaline is, therefore, absolutely essential. This is repeated, according to response, every 10–15 minutes. Where the antigen contact has occurred at a single, accessible site (e.g. a bee sting on the arm), 100–300 μg adrenaline injected subcutaneously at the site may slow antigen absorption. Patients who have a predominantly airway response may benefit from inhaled adrenaline, but injectable adrenaline should be used promptly if there is no improvement within 2 minutes of the inhalation of two puffs (child) or four puffs (adult) of adrenaline from pMDI.

Adrenaline given intravenously is associated with a number of very unpleasant effects (**Fig. 5.12**). It should, therefore, be administered in this way *only* in very severe cases (where there is total vascular shutdown), as 400–500 μg adrenaline, given over a period of 3 minutes. Unless cardiac monitoring and full resuscitation skills and facilities are available, the risks of this route may outweigh the benefits.

A good response to adrenaline can confirm the diagnosis of anaphylactic reaction. Part of the follow-up to treatment is therefore to ask the patient 'Did the adrenaline make you feel better?'

maintain respiration with oxygen, inhaled bronchodilator, and/or intravenous aminophylline

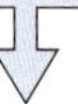

If there is no immediate response to the adrenaline, oxygen can be given, either by nasal 'spectacles' or by face mask. The patency of the airway should be assured, by intubation (**Fig. 5.13**) or even by tracheotomy if necessary. Assisted ventilation may be necessary at this point.

Bronchospasm that is unrelieved despite adrenaline treatment can be treated with inhaled bronchodilator (e.g. salbutamol administered by pMDI or nebulizer), or by infusion of intravenous aminophylline (10–20 ml of aminophylline 250 mg/10 ml at a rate of 2 ml/minute).

Use of adrenaline in anaphylaxis	
administration:	intramuscular injection (intravenous route is for emergency use only, where cardiac resuscitation is required)
side-effects:	anxiety tremor tachycardia arrhythmias dry mouth cold extremities
possible interactions with:	anaesthetics antidepressants beta-blockers other sympathomimetics, e.g. dopexamine

Fig. 5.12 Use of adrenaline in anaphylaxis. Adverse effects can be particularly severe when the drug is administered intravenously.

restore circulation with crystalloid

The vasopermeability and decreased vascular resistance caused by anaphylaxis and extravasation leads to vascular pooling with a rise in haematocrit and increased blood viscosity, manifesting in the patient as hypotension or shock. This volume should be replaced as a matter of urgency with crystalloid or, if available, with colloid.

Persistent hypotension may require the use of alpha-adrenergic agents, such as dopamine. Where these drugs are used, cardiac rhythm and blood pressure should be carefully monitored.

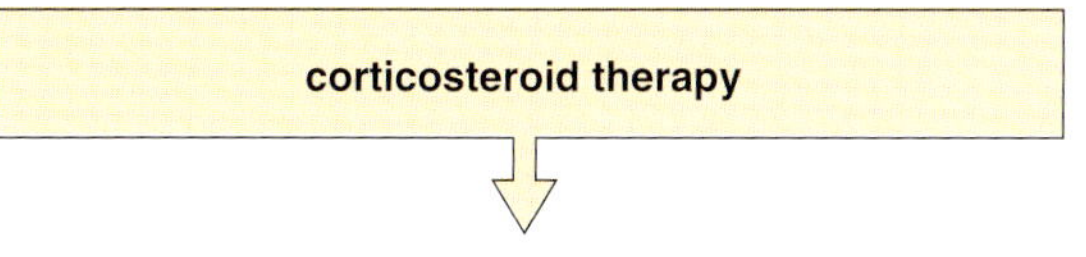

corticosteroid therapy

There is no evidence that corticosteroids, with their relatively slow onset of action, have any effect on the course of acute reactions. However, the possibility of late relapse of anaphylactic reactions seems to justify their use. They may be administered orally, intramuscularly, or intravenously. As with antihistamines, the condition of the patient will dictate the route of administration. Although intravenous hydrocortisone can exacerbate the anaphylactic reaction in aspirin-sensitive asthmatics, this may be the only possible route if the patient is critically ill.

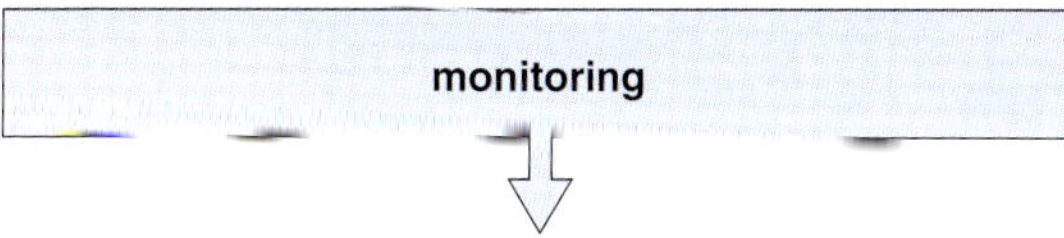

monitoring

The risk of relapse, due to a prolonged or biphasic reaction, or to the re-establishment of symptoms once the relatively short-lived effects of adrenaline have passed, means that the patient should be closely monitored for at least 6–8 hours, or at least until it is certain that the condition has stabilized. Admission to hospital may be necessary if the patient's condition is severe.

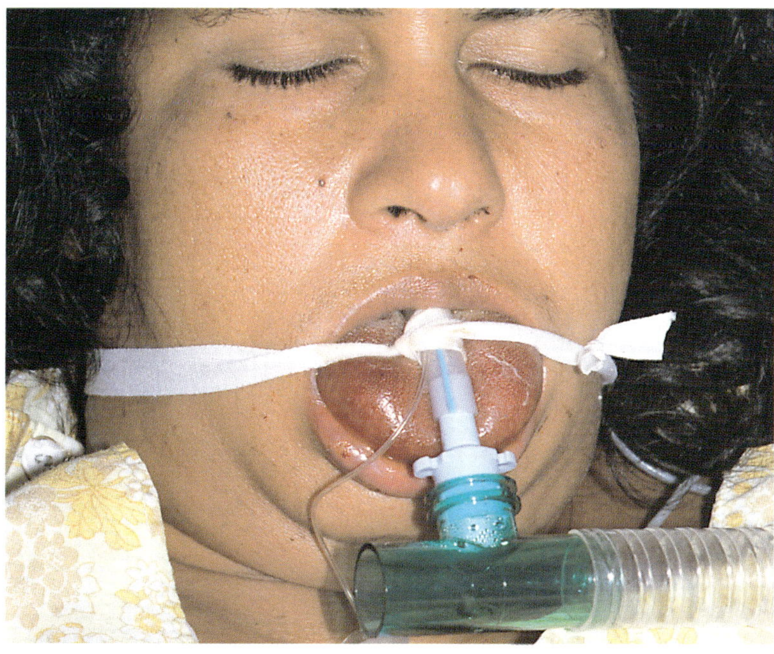

Fig. 5.13 Severe angioedema in a 43-year-old woman. She required endotracheal intubation to overcome laryngeal obstruction. Note the oedema of her mouth and face.

education and prevention

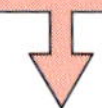

Identify and avoid precipitants

Because anaphylactic reactions normally occur almost immediately after exposure to the precipitating antigen, this agent is usually easily identified. Where the cause is in doubt – for example where the agent is one of several drugs given simultaneously – then referral to a specialist may be necessary. Identification may require re-challenge, a procedure that requires the presence of resuscitation facilities and staff.

Patients should be advised assiduously to avoid precipitating factors. This can be straightforward, but may be difficult when the agent is covertly present in foods, as is the case with peanuts for example (**Fig. 5.14**), or when the agent is an important drug.

It may not be possible to entirely eliminate the precipitating agent from the patient's surroundings. For example, patients demonstrating anaphylactic reaction to bee or wasp stings should reduce the risk of contact as far as possible by avoiding settings where the insects are likely to congregate, for example.

Patients should also be aware of the possibility of cross-reactions – a reaction against aspirin may mean that all NSAIDs should be avoided – and should modify their behaviour accordingly.

Tests

Tests for patients with anaphylactic reactions come in three forms: skin tests, blood tests, and challenge tests.

Skin tests can be either prick tests or intradermal tests. The latter are performed only in hospitals, as the sensitivity is 100- to 1000-fold greater than that achiev-

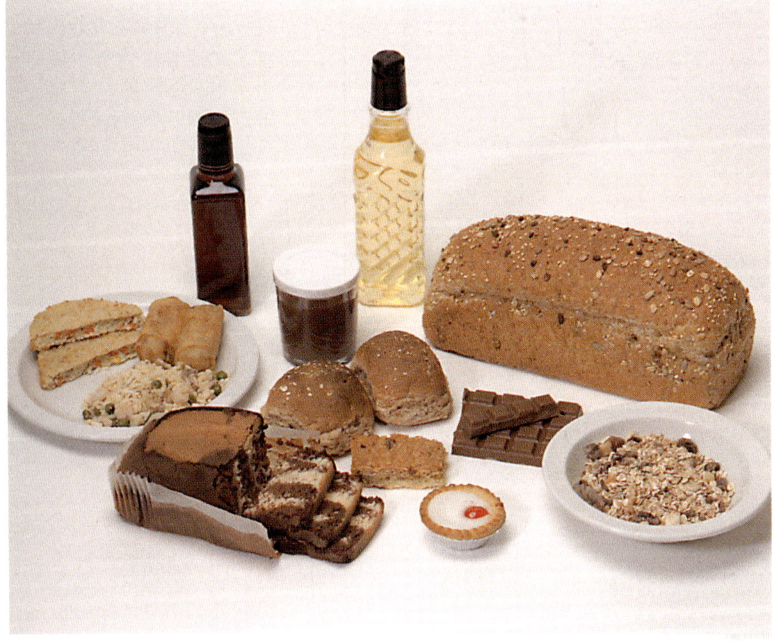

Fig. 5.14 Some foods which may contain peanut.

able with a prick test. It is therefore usual to perform the prick test first. If the result is negative then the intradermal method will be considered. Skin tests are useful for venoms, some drugs (e.g. muscle relaxants, and antibiotics), and foods (*see* Chapter 6). False positive skin reactions can be a problem, as some drugs are histamine releasers in their own right, with high concentrations precipitating non-specific reactions. Other drugs (e.g. NSAIDs) will give false negative reactions. The difficulties of testing for drug allergy are exemplified in the design of the recently introduced 'Allergopen kit', designed to identify penicillin allergy. The kit contains samples of the drug (the 'major determinant'), as well as the products of penicillin polymerization and degradation (the 'minor determinant mixture'), two processes that can occur when the drug is stored.

Few *in vitro* (blood) tests exist for the detection of drug sensitivity. However, a new generation of blood tests are currently in development. They work by measuring the release of mediators from basophils, and offer promise for the future.

Challenge testing is often the only way to identify a trigger factor when all other tests have given a negative result. For example, aspirin sensitivity, often overlooked by skin testing, can be elicited following the inhalation of lysine aspirin, a derivative suitable for the inhaled route.

Know how to deal with attacks

Any patient with a history of attacks should carry some form of identification, such as a MedicAlert bracelet, at all times.

Where the subject is a child, it is particularly important that teachers and other potential carers have an emergency management plan for the treatment of anaphylactic shock. All such materials should be simple but comprehensive (**Figs 5.15 & 5.16**)

Anaphylactic shock: what to look for
Urticarial rash (nettle rash/hives) pale pink and raised, intensely itchy
Flushed face and neck
Swollen lips and tongue
Hoarse voice and/or noisy breathing
Difficulty breathing and/or difficulty swallowing
Feeling of faintness and/or apprehension
Loss of consciousness
Rapid weak pulse
Very laboured breathing
Blue colour to the lips

Fig. 5.15 Anaphylactic shock: what to look for. A checklist for parents, guardians and schoolteachers of the signs of impending anaphylaxis.

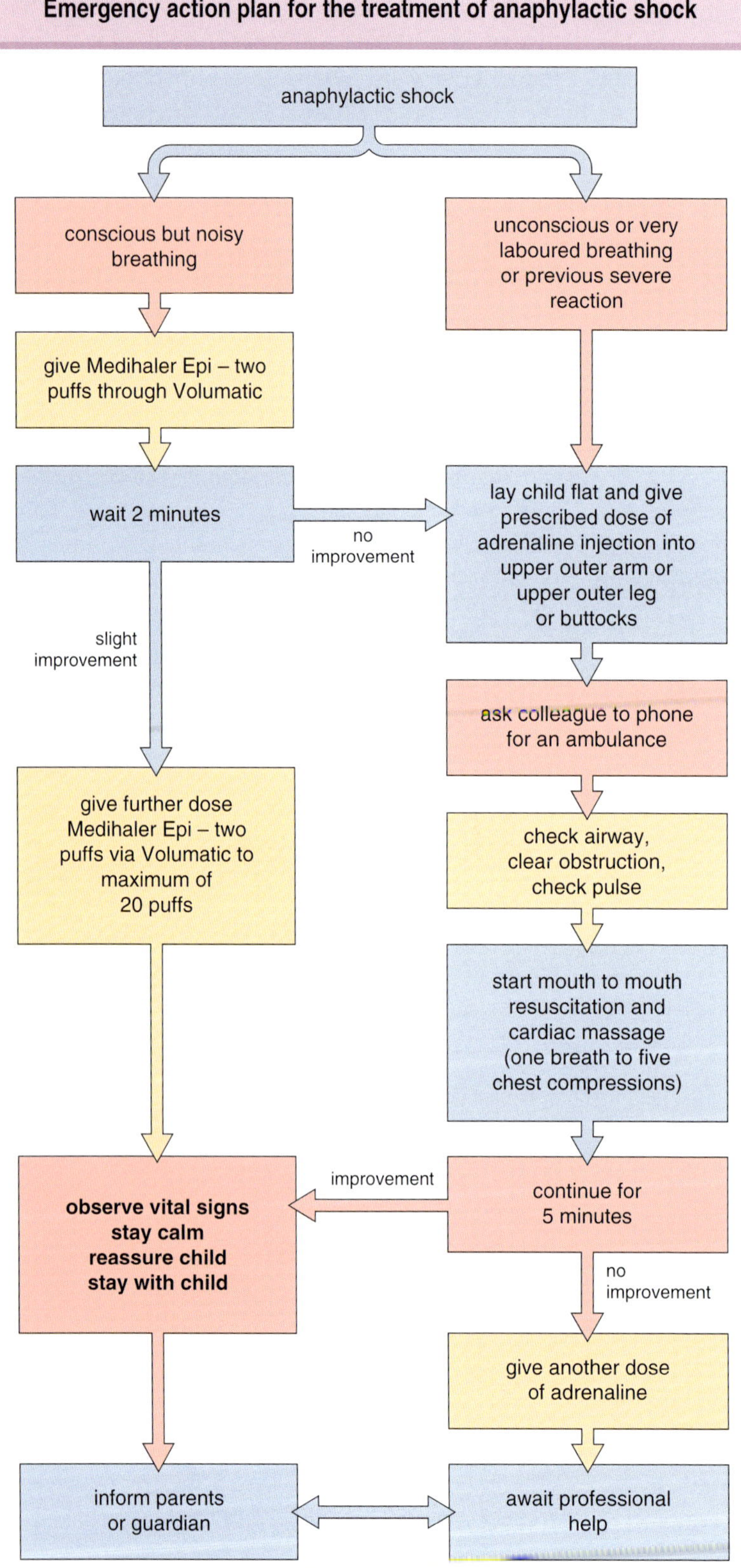

Fig. 5.16 Emergency action plan for the treatment of anaphylactic shock. This plan is designed principally for the use of schoolteachers where a child is known to be at risk. For the plan to be useful, it must use the correct tradenames for the various drugs and devices.

Adrenaline should be kept at the patient's home, and other family members should be instructed in its use. Patients who have a predominantly airway response can use inhaled adrenaline, but others will need to administer it subcutaneously. Syringes, always difficult for the novice to manipulate under conditions of stress, have been superseded by the adrenaline pen. A range of models are now available, and all are easy to use (**Fig. 5.17**). Two should be kept in the house at all times.

Does every patient with a history of anaphylactic reaction, no matter how mild, need an adrenaline pen? The answer to this is that it is impossible to be sure. On average, the best predictor of the severity of the next reaction is the severity of the last one. However, a mild reaction can be followed by death on the next attack, and a near fatal attack can just as easily be followed by a mild case of urticaria. Patients with risk factors such as asthma, old age with hypertension, ischaemic heart disease or cerebral insufficiency need particular consideration as they form the main group at risk of fatal reaction.

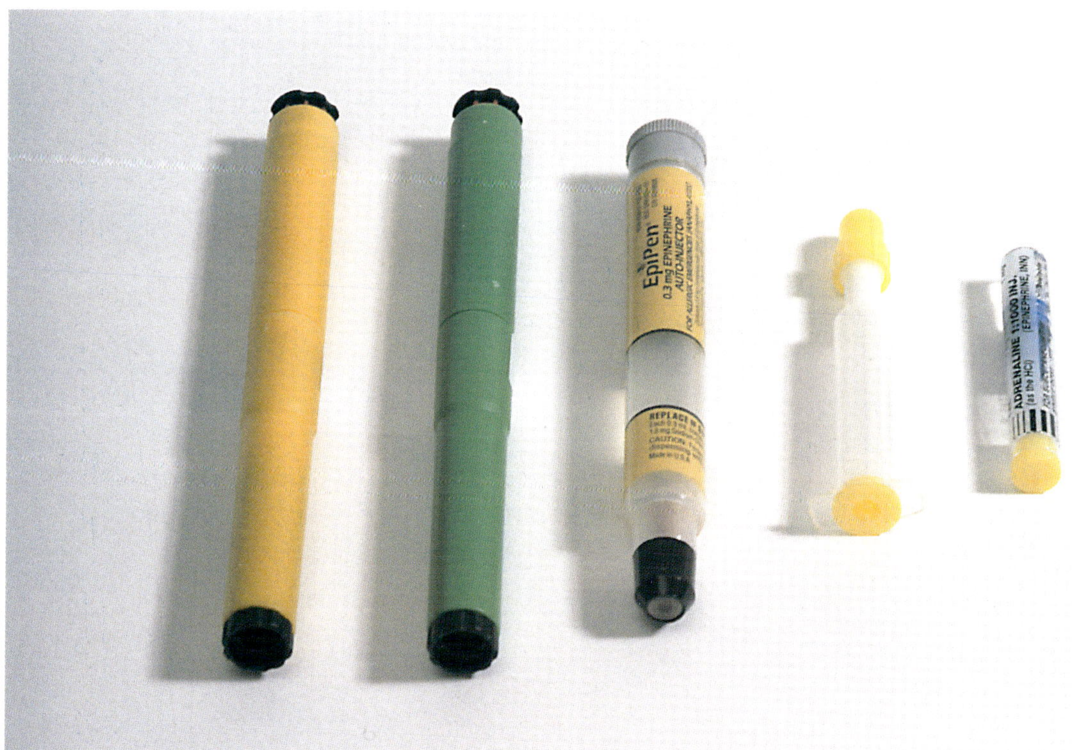

Fig. 5.17 A selection of adrenaline pens.

Desensitization

Where the precipitating agent is hard to avoid, and if the resulting reaction is likely to be life threatening, a course of desensitizing therapy can be undertaken. This is possible, for example, in patients allergic to bee and wasp stings.

The method is to subject the patient to increasingly large doses of the antigen over a period of days or weeks, followed by maintenance at the top dose for 2–3 years. This is a potentially dangerous procedure, and must be carried out under controlled conditions with resuscitation equipment, and staff skilled in its use, on standby (**Fig. 5.18**).

Selection of patients for immunotherapy can only be made by specialists. Patients with a history of hypotension, collapse, urticaria, laryngeal oedema, or asthma following a sting should be referred by the GP or casualty officer for assessment.

Patients accepted for the procedure are likely to have a history of one or more moderate-to-severe systemic reactions, and a positive skin-prick test or RAST to venom.

Doses are usually given every 4 weeks initially, with the period increasing to 4–6 weeks once the maintenance dose has been reached. If these maintenance doses are not administered at the correct intervals the protection will wane. The optimum treatment period is probably three years, but therapy can be discontinued sooner if RAST and skin tests are negative, and remain negative.

In the case of drug-induced anaphylaxis, patients with reactivity to drugs needed for their effective treatment can also be desensitized by the rising dose method, treating adverse reactions as they arise. However, the tolerance induced continues only as long as the drug continues to be administered.

The safety record of desensitization therapy is excellent. Patients with hypertension or angina and patients taking beta-blockers have all been successfully desensitized.

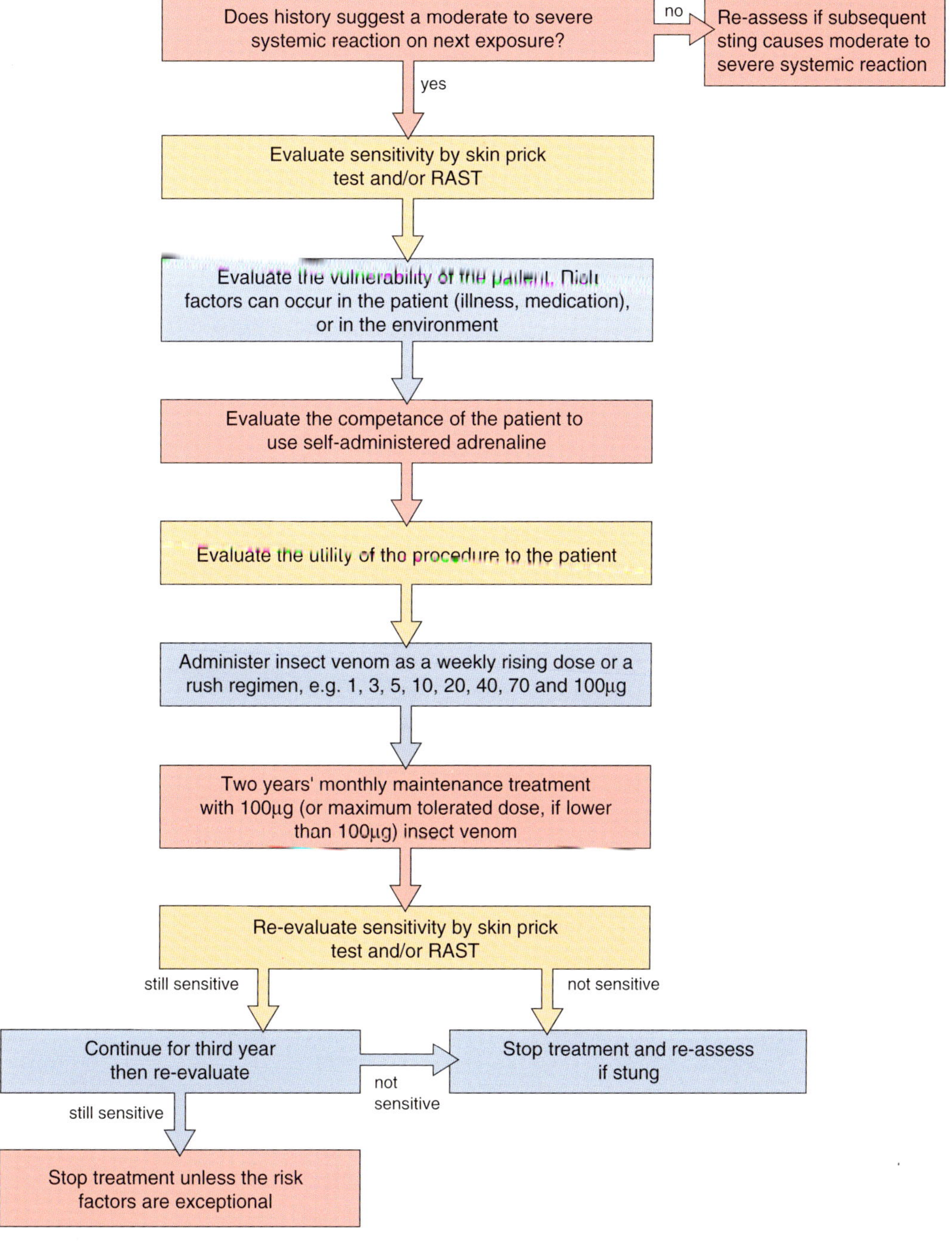

Fig. 5.18 Protocol for venom immunotherapy (desensitization).

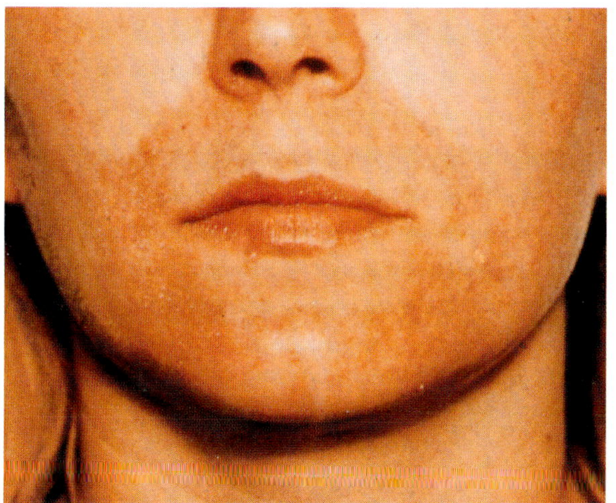
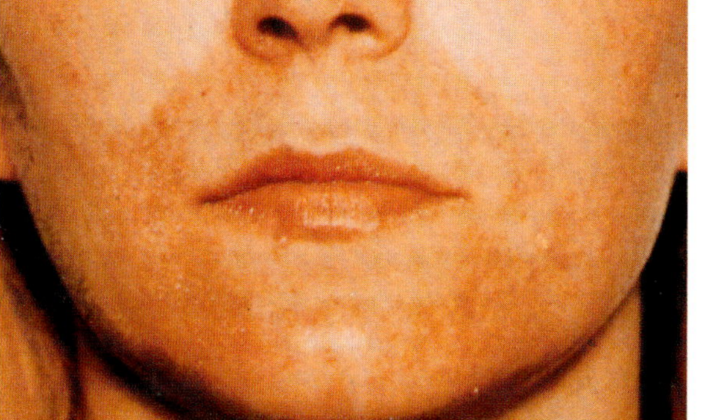

Fig 6.5 Perioral eczema. The perioral distribution of the lesions suggested a contact or ingested cause, and the patient suspected an orange drink to be the cause. Citrus fruits are among the commoner causes of food-related symptoms, but in this case the food colourings tartrazine (E102) and sunset yellow (E110) were responsible, and were identified by exclusion diet.

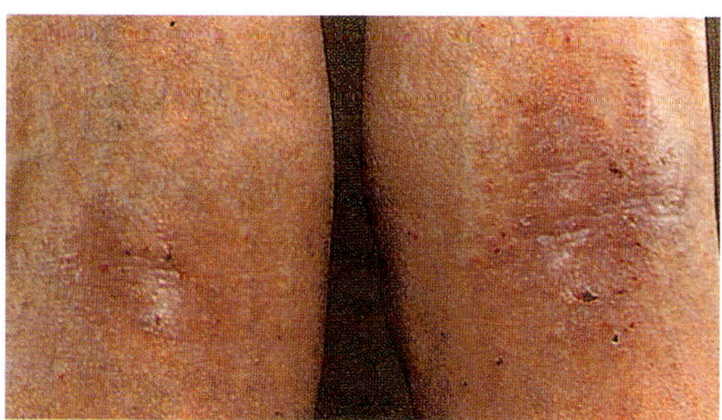

Fig 6.6 A 2-year-old girl with atopic eczema. Note the extensive dermatitis in the knee flexures. At this stage, some children show an improvement if cow's milk, egg, or other substances are eliminated from their diet. However, atopic eczema is rarely – if ever – due to food allergy alone.

distinguish food intolerance from food allergy

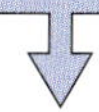

Food-related medical history

As in many other areas of clinical medicine, the importance of a careful medical history cannot be overemphasized (**Fig. 6.7**). As well as taking a full personal and family history, it is helpful to ask about factors that may have been associated with the onset of the condition. These could include viral illnesses, broad-spectrum antibiotic therapy (particularly when prolonged or recurrent), and major emotional stresses.

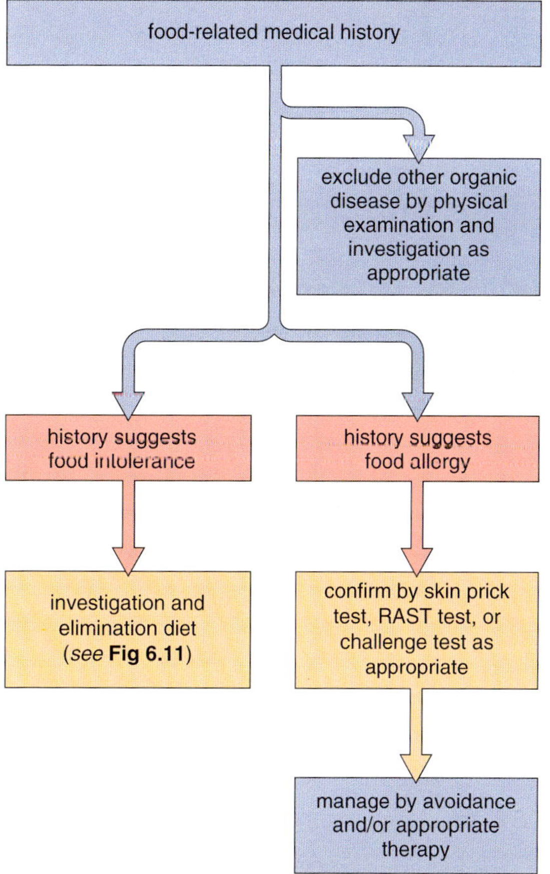

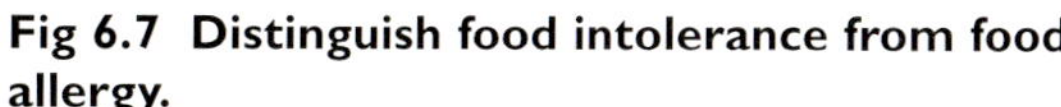

Fig 6.7 Distinguish food intolerance from food allergy.

Exclude other organic disease by physical examination and investigation as appropriate

Before investigating food hypersensitivity phenomena, careful physical examination and investigation is important. It is all too easy to overlook other polysymptomatic conditions, such as occult carcinoma, collagen diseases and chronic infections, that can mimic food intolerance.

History suggests food allergy

An immediate hypersensitivity reaction to a particular food is often clearly apparent to the patient. Supporting evidence from the medical history includes a family and personal history of atopic disease. Conditions in which such reactions are likely to be encountered are listed in **Fig. 6.1**.

Difficulties may arise when a consistent trigger food cannot be identified by the patient. In this situation it may be helpful to show the patient a list of foods known to be capable of producing immediate food hypersensitivity reactions. Note that some trigger foods are present as ingredients of proprietary foods, or are eaten in quantities so small as to seem irrelevant to the patient (e.g. sesame seed on bread). A food diary may help the patient to identify the cause of the reaction. The temptation to classify the problem as 'idiopathic' should be resisted until all possible food triggers have been examined.

Food-related anaphylaxis may be brought on by strenuous exercise taken immediately after eating. This condition (food-dependent exercise-induced anaphylaxis, or FDEIA) has been described in relationship to celery, shellfish and wheat in specifically sensitized individuals. Unexplained (non-specific) FDEIA episodes, where any food can act as the co-trigger, are occasionally seen.

Confirm by skin prick test, radioallergosorbent test, or challenge test as appropriate

Skin prick tests and RASTs are useful when they support the clinical history. However, it is not unusual to see an immediate clinical hypersensitivity response to a specific food in the absence of positive SPT or RAST. Consideration should then be given to performing the SPT with a small quantity of fresh food (a freshly squeezed drop of juice, or a few crumbs 'puddled' in saline), in case the commercial extract has given a false-negative response.

Support for the existence of immediate oral reactions to food (the oral allergy syndrome) is provided by the finding of positive SPT or RAST results to a related food or pollen. Cross-reactivities between food and non-food antigens have been identified, and in some cases the common chemical antigen has been determined (**Fig. 6.8**). Knowledge of these relationships can help both

Cross-reacting groups of plant-derived allergens	
Non-food	**Food**
Pollen	
Silver birch, Hazel, Hornbeam, Mugwort	Parsnip, orange, raw apple, onion, raw carrot, tomato, potato, hazelnut, raw celery
Grasses	Peach, apricot, nectarine, plum, cherry
Compositae (daisy family)	Sunflower seeds, lychee
Latex (contact)	Banana, avocado, chestnut, kiwi fruit, pineapple

Fig 6.8 Cross-reacting groups of plant-derived allergens. The foods involved commonly co-present as triggers of oral allergy syndrome, often with evidence of associated allergic reaction to non-food plant allergens (e.g. latex or pollen).

doctor and patient to identify the cause of the hypersensitivity reaction.

Challenge tests are seldom required to confirm immediate food hypersensitivity. They should be be used only when avoidance of the suspect food is likely to be difficult, and where the allergy cannot be confirmed by either RAST or SPT. Challenge tests should be carried out with resuscitation facilities immediately available. The elucidation of FDEIA in this way presents an exacting challenge to the investigator.

Manage by avoidance and/or appropriate therapy

Where possible, the allergen should be avoided in food allergy, as in other allergic disorders. With allergy to a single food substance, this is sometimes possible. However, some common allergens, such as peanut, are widely distributed in prepared foods and even the most thorough avoidance techniques may fail.

Additional treatment in food allergy depends on the symptom complex induced by the allergic reaction and follows the principles outlined in other chapters of this book. Patients with urticaria, angioedema or the oral allergy syndrome may benefit from the immediate use of an antihistamine at the first hint of symptoms. Patients who are known to be at risk of asthma must be given appropriate therapy (*see* Chapters 2–4), and those with potentially life-threatening reactions, such as laryngeal oedema and anaphylaxis, must carry and be trained in the use of inhalable or injectable adrenaline (*see* Chapter 5).

History suggests food intolerance

It is not uncommon for patients to believe that some part of their diet is responsible for their illness, and psychologically based food aversion may result. Such cases should be resolved in a responsible and clear-cut manner. Both doctor and patient must be satisfied that food is not causing the illness. It is equally important to identify genuine food intolerance reactions so that appropriate treatment can be given and unnecessary suffering can be avoided. It is inappropriate to dismiss the possibility of food intolerance simply because SPT and/or RAST results to a wide range of foods are negative.

Foods associated with immediate hypersensitivity reactions are often correctly identified by the patient at presentation. However, foods causing non-immediate reactions usually go unsuspected, while some patients will incorrectly identify harmless foods as triggers.

Clues in the history which suggest non-immediate food hypersensitivity include the following:

- Symptoms are often multiple and relate to a number of different systems (**Fig. 6.9**).
- Symptoms are typically recurrent or episodic. When there is a marked regular pattern of diurnal variation, intolerance of a staple food (e.g. milk, wheat, corn, egg) may be suspected. However, the occurrence of episodic symptoms (e.g. migraine occurring once a month) does not mean that the implicated food is only eaten at this frequency.

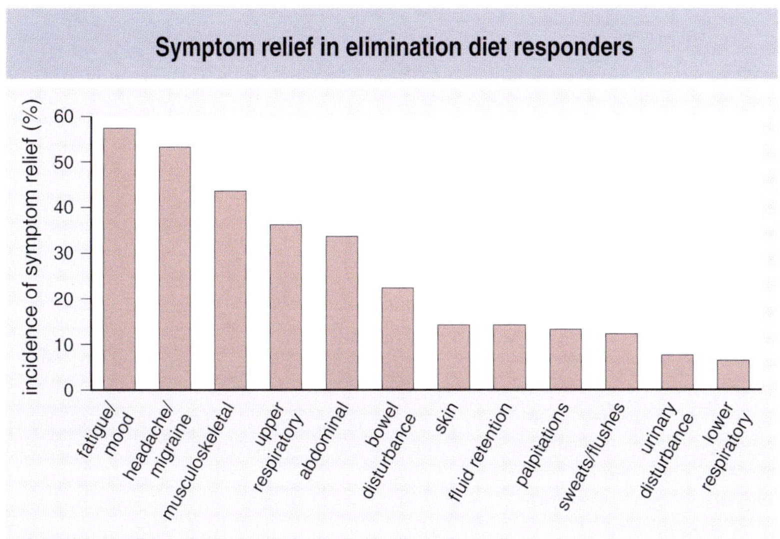

Fig 6.9 Symptom relief in elimination diet responders. Data from Radcliffe MJ. Clinical methods for diagnosis. *Clin Immunol Allergy* 1982; **2**: 205–20.

- The patient may know that he is upset by the food in one form, and yet still be eating it in other forms. Thus, he may not be able to drink milk, but regularly eats cheese or yoghurt. Staple foods (e.g. wheat, maize, milk, yeast, egg and soya) are often found as 'hidden' ingredients in processed foods, and are therefore particularly difficult to avoid.
- The patient is sometimes unusually habituated to the implicated food and may feel inexplicably threatened by the idea that he should now avoid it (this is very rare in food allergy).
- Symptoms may be precipitated by the omission of an implicated staple food, and relieved by its consumption. This inversion of the expected response has been termed 'masking'. For example, the migraine that typically occurs when breakfast is omitted may be related to intolerance of a breakfast food such as wheat. Similarly, the patient complaining of unexplained fatigue who gets a 'lift' from drinking milk may be suffering a masked reaction to it. For this reason, the patient's answer to the question 'What food makes you feel better?' can be illuminating. It is possible that such reactions relate to the presence of biologically active peptides with morphine-like activity (exorphins) in the implicated foods. (Opiates are known to possess the capacity to release histamine from mast cells.)

withdraw non-essential medication, do symptom scores, and measure baseline parameters

A baseline record of symptoms can be made on a diary card. This can include any self-measurable parameter of disease activity, e.g. peak flow rate, severity of skin disorder (**Fig. 6.10**). The baseline period should be sufficient to give a general measure of the level and frequency of usually encountered symptoms. The diary card should ideally be continued over the period of the elimination diet.

Orally administered medications usually contain food-related items as excipients. Food starches are commonly used as fillers (e.g. corn, soya or potato starch in tablets). Liquid medicines may contain food as sweeteners (e.g. corn syrup). For all but the simplest of elimination diets, non-essential medications should therefore be withdrawn or replaced with alternatives known to be free from the excipient items.

For the same reason, toothpaste should be avoided and replaced with a simple tooth powder made from 50:50 sodium chloride and sodium bicarbonate. This is more palatable if finely ground, for example in a well cleaned coffee grinder. A couple of drops of oil of peppermint may be added if desired.

Recording food intolerance

	Week 1 Mon	Tue	Wed	Thu	Fri	Sat	Sun	Week 2 Mon	Tue	Wed	Thu	Fri	Sat	Sun	Week 3 Mon
0 : nil 1 : mild 2 : moderate 3 : severe 4 : very severe main symptoms															
1															
2															
3															
4															
5															
6															

etc

Fig 6.10 Recording food intolerance. This chart serves to record symptom scores at all stages of the investigation: pre-elimination, elimination, and individual sequential food challenge.

progressive elimination diet to establish the remission of symptoms

The next step is to achieve remission of symptoms by means of an elimination diet (**Fig. 6.11**).

Specific elimination of certain foods and/or food additives

It may be tempting to begin by eliminating only food additives from the diet, or by avoiding just one or two common foods. There are a number of drawbacks to this approach, severely limiting the chance of success. Most sufferers of food intolerance are sensitive to more than one item, and even when there are clues to the main food item responsible, a negative response is often caused by missing an associated trigger food. Another common reason for failure is the fact that an increasing number of foods are used as 'hidden' ingredients by the food industry (**Fig. 6.12**). As a result the patient may fail to completely exclude the food under test.

Broad-based elimination diet (e.g. 'stone-age diet')

In practice it is simpler to set a diet that indicates what can be eaten, rather than what should be avoided. This

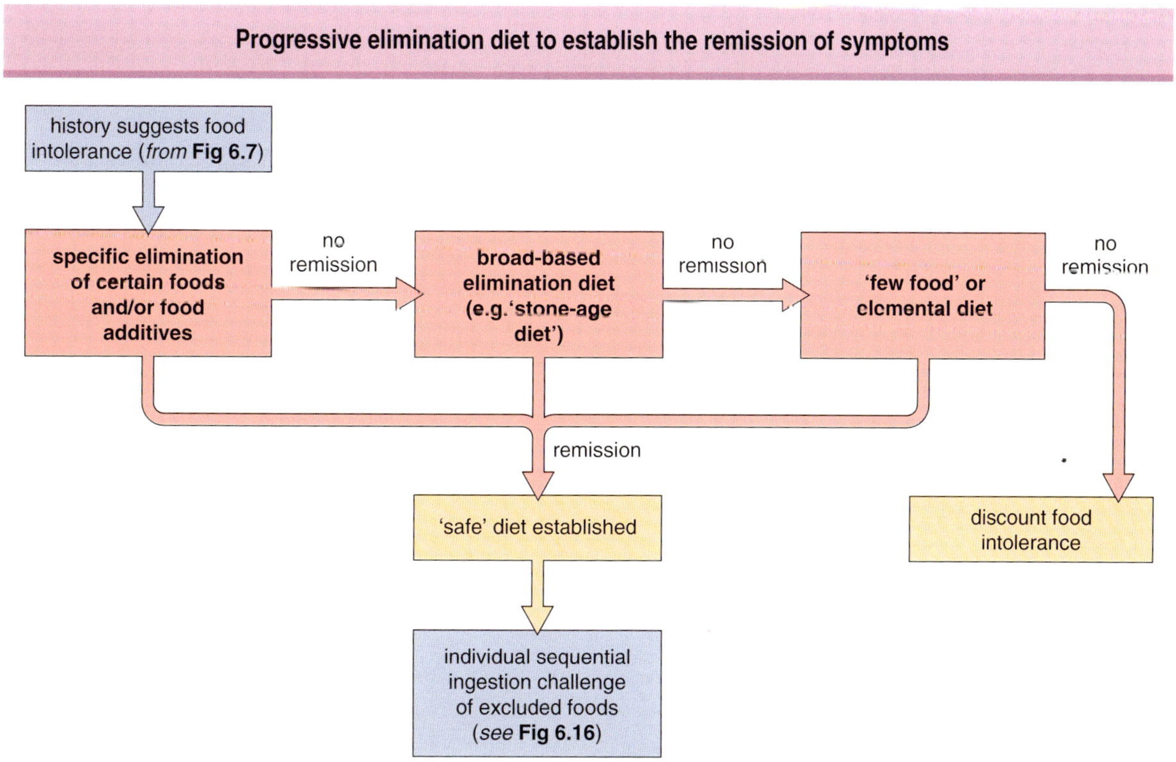

Progressive elimination diet to establish the remission of symptoms

history suggests food intolerance (*from* **Fig 6.7**)

specific elimination of certain foods and/or food additives

no remission

broad-based elimination diet (e.g.'stone-age diet')

no remission

'few food' or elemental diet

no remission

remission

'safe' diet established

discount food intolerance

individual sequential ingestion challenge of excluded foods (*see* **Fig 6.16**)

Fig 6.11 Progressive elimination diet to establish the remission of symptoms.

Hidden foods	
Food	**May be contained in:**
Milk	Foods labelled with casein, caseinate, lactose and whey Powdered artificial sweeteners 'Non-dairy' milk and cream substitutes Bread Margarine Ice cream (even labelled 'contains non-milk fat') Sausages, hamburgers *Plain* chocolate Sherbet, other sweets
Egg	Foods labelled with vitellin, ovovitellin, livetin, ovomucin, ovomucoid and albumin Unlabelled in baking powder, cakes, croissants, glazed bread/rolls, pastry, meringue Sauces Salad dressings Icing, sweets Sausages, luncheon meats Wines, coffee and root beer
Wheat	Foods labelled starch, food starch, germ, bran and farina Gluten-free flour (not all is completely wheat-free) Baking powder Sausages Vinegar Alcoholic beverages Rye (the seed may be up to 10% wheat contaminated)

Fig 6.12 Hidden foods. An increasing number of common foods occur as hidden ingredients in manufactured foods. Sometimes the presence of such foods is apparent from the label. However this is not always the case.

largely avoids the risk of hidden ingredients, and although the diet may be restrictive, patients find it easier to follow (**Fig. 6.13**).

The biggest problem for the average patient will be finding substitutes for tea, coffee, and bread. Buckwheat pancakes can replace bread where absolutely necessary (e.g. in packed lunches) and are relatively easy to prepare.

'Few food' and elemental diets

The 'few food' diet is more restrictive, but for many patients is no more difficult to follow than a broad-based elimination diet. It is based on foods known to be unlikely to produce intolerance (**Fig. 6.14**). It is vitally important to remember that even a highly restrictive elimination diet may fail if the diet happens to include a problem food.

An elemental diet consists of a well-balanced, residue-free mixture of amino acids, simple sugars, electrolytes, trace elements and vitamins. Such diets are capable of supporting nutritional intake over a long period of time while waiting for a remission. However, they may retain an intolerance-producing capacity and are not popular with patients.

Remission

Whichever elimination diet is used, withdrawal effects are often (but not always) encountered, particularly in the case of withdrawal of non-tolerated staple foods. Typically these withdrawal effects will commence on the afternoon or evening of the first day. Common early withdrawal effects include headache, which is often migrainous, agitation and depression. The effects of withdrawal of a problem food are analagous to those associated with the withdrawal of alcohol, drugs, caffeine and tobacco.

Late withdrawal effects include myalgia and fatigue. Patients often describe their symptoms as 'just like flu without the fever'. Tachycardia with minimal exertion is common on the second, third or fourth day. Such symptoms may lead the sufferer to break the diet, inappropriately ascribing symptoms to hunger rather than to withdrawal effects. However, these symptoms are temporary and quickly disappear.

With or without a withdrawal phase, symptom clearance is usually apparent by the fifth to tenth day of the elimination phase. To provide adequate evidence of remission, however, it is sometimes necessary to continue the diet. The remission of symptoms is often dramatic, but must be sufficiently prolonged, taking into account baseline frequency and severity, so as to be unequivocal.

A broad-based elimination diet	
Fresh meat	Any kind including offal
Fresh fish	Any kind
Fresh vegetables	Any kind except potato and tomato (yam or sweet potato can be substituted for potato)
Fresh fruit	Any kind except citrus
Grain	Rice, rice cakes, rice noodles
Grain substitute	Buckwheat, quinoa
Drinks	Spring water, additive-free juices of allowed fruit, herb and fruit teas (e.g. mint, rosehip, rooibosch, ruby red)
Seasoning	Sea salt, fresh pepper and herbs
Oils	Olive, sunflower, safflower (avoid unidentified vegetable oil)

Fig 6.13 A broad-based elimination diet. This may be modified under certain circumstances (e.g. if allergy to fruits is suspected)

A 'few foods' diet		
Cod	Swede	Courgette
Trout	Sweet potato	Carrot
Mackerel	Quinoa	Peach
Pear	Celery	Safflower oil
Avocado pear	Bean sprouts	Sea salt
Parsnip	Marrow	Olive oil

Fig 6.14 A 'few foods' diet. These foods are amongst the least likely to produce non-immediate hypersensitivity (food intolerance). However, it should be noted that celery and carrot (especially when uncooked) are foods capable of producing immediate food hypersensitivity (food allergy).

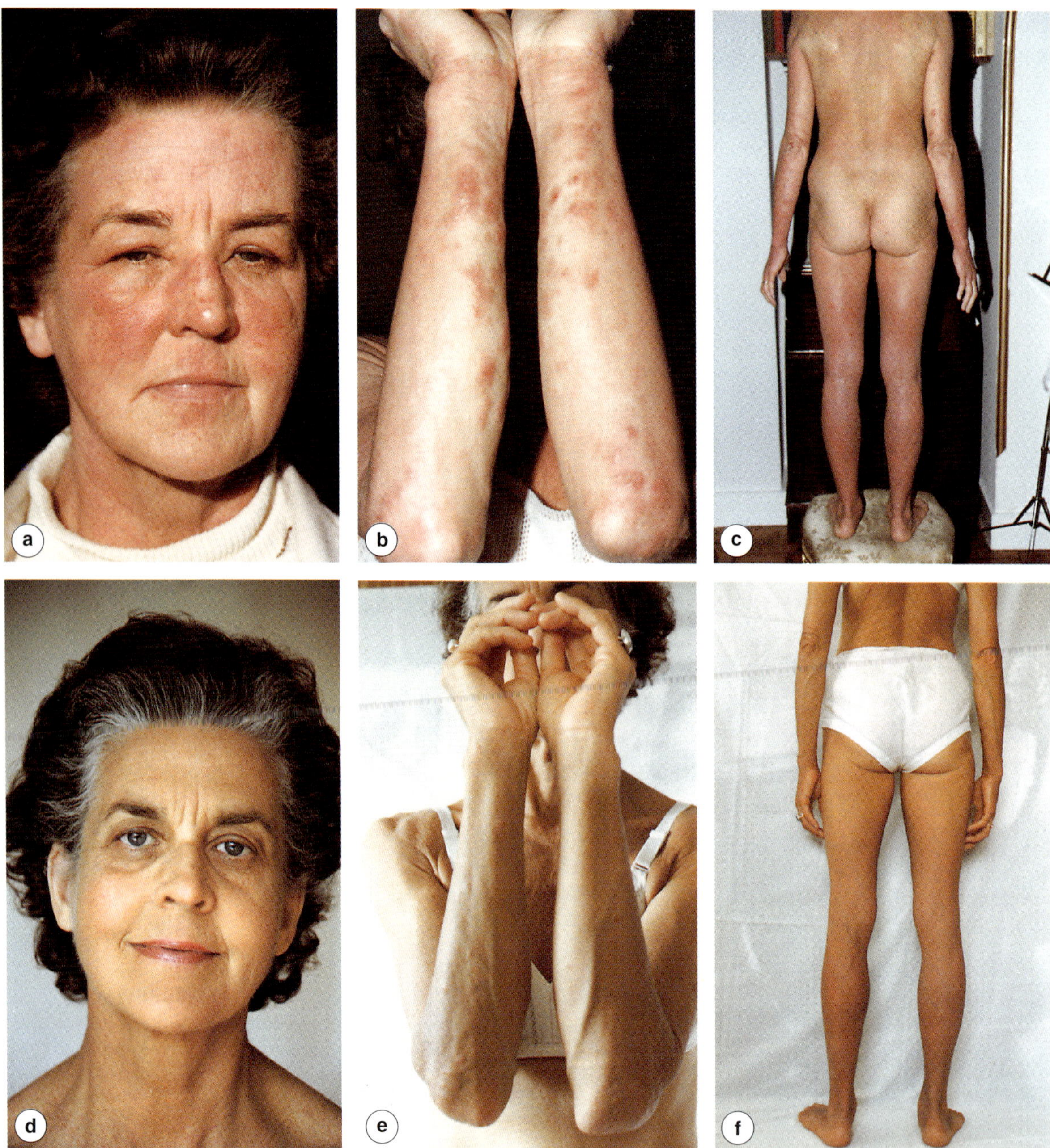

Fig 6.15 A woman aged 58 years had a history of asthma since childhood. In her late 40s the asthma had become less troublesome and less persistent, but she developed severe eczema. She became dependent on fluorinated steroid creams. During an attack of gastroenteritis, she underwent a fast for a few days and the eczema briefly cleared. A while later, she experienced a particularly troublesome exfoliative phase and became severely depressed. She decided to further investigate the connection with diet. For eight weeks she followed a personalized 'few foods' diet, used dust mite control measures and changed her clothes to cotton or silk. There was no improvement in the eczema (a–c). In desperation she reduced her diet to three foods only (lamb, cabbage and carrot) and her eczema cleared completely over the next month (d–f). Sequential food challenge subsequently identified numerous trigger foods and defined a test-negative diet. The reactive foods in the 'few foods' diet proved in retrospect to be rice and onion. She has now been in complete remission for 2 years controlled by diet alone. There has been no recurrence of her asthma.

No remission

Lack of full symptom remission should lead one to ask whether all responsible foods have been eliminated. It is easy to draw a false-negative conclusion from an elimination regime which was either itself inadequate, or was applied without adequate attention to detail (**Fig. 6.15**).

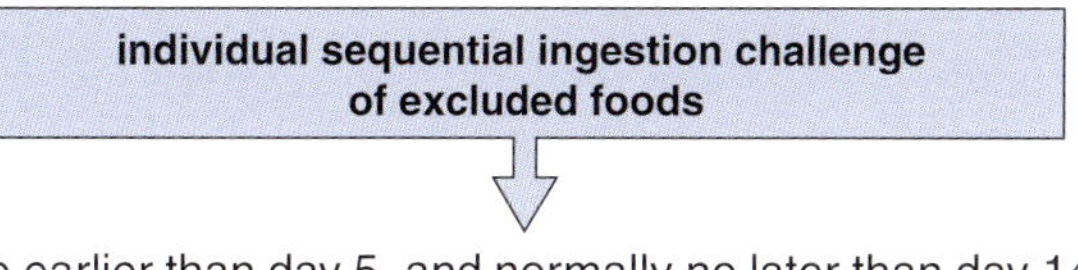

No earlier than day 5, and normally no later than day 14 of the elimination diet, assuming that there has been a clearance of both pre-existing and withdrawal symptoms, sequential food ingestion challenge testing can begin (**Fig. 6.16**). Foods to be tested should be eaten alone and unadulterated. For example, use wheat (e.g. Shredded Wheat) rather than bread, pure cocoa powder rather than chocolate, and black tea rather than tea with milk.

The way in which a food is prepared can determine whether or not a patient is reactive to it. Foods should therefore be eaten in all forms normally encountered by the patient. For example, when testing tomato, both raw and cooked tomato should be eaten together.

Foods to be tested should be those commonly eaten by the patient. As a minimum, any food that has been eliminated, and that is usually consumed by the patient more often than once a week, should be tested. In

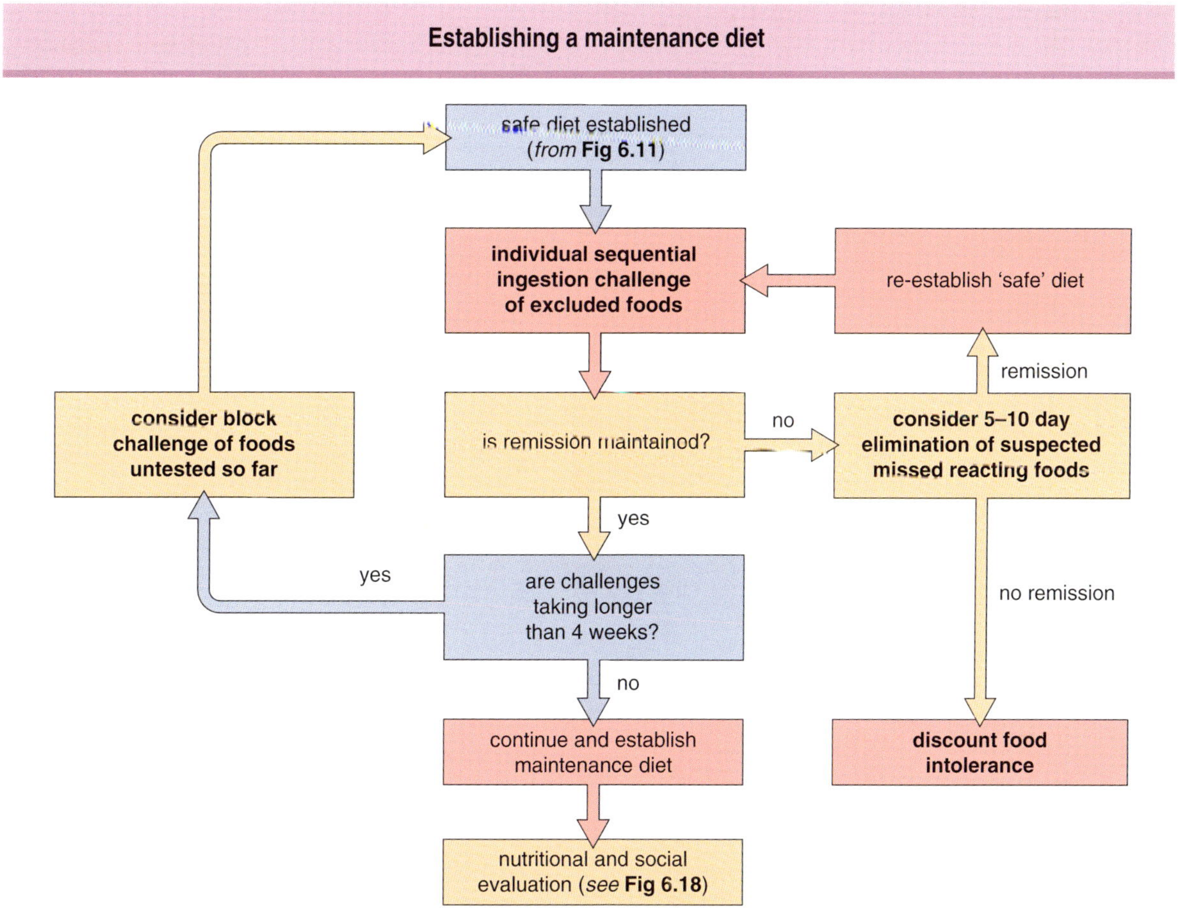

Establishing a maintenance diet

safe diet established (*from* **Fig 6.11**)

individual sequential ingestion challenge of excluded foods

re-establish 'safe' diet

remission

consider block challenge of foods untested so far

is remission maintained?

no

consider 5–10 day elimination of suspected missed reacting foods

yes

yes

are challenges taking longer than 4 weeks?

no remission

no

continue and establish maintenance diet

discount food intolerance

nutritional and social evaluation (*see* **Fig 6.18**)

Fig 6.16 Establishing a maintenance diet.

particular the following commonly implicated foods, many of which are contained as 'hidden' ingredients of commercially prepared foods, should be tested (**Fig. 6.17**): wheat, milk, egg, corn, potato, coffee, tea, soya, yeast, chocolate, citrus fruit, and cheese.

If the patient's routine allows it, food testing can be done either at breakfast time or at lunch time. If no symptoms occur, the food can be added to the evening meal of 'safe' foods. Provided there are no symptoms by the next morning, another food test can be conducted the next day.

The results of food tests should be recorded by the patient using the same format that was used for symptom recording during the elimination diet (see **Fig. 6.6**). An increase in heart rate is common in the hour following re-introduction of a non-tolerated food. Some physicians therefore record the pulse before the challenge, and 20, 40 and 60 minutes after it.

Masked reactions to foods

The technique of food elimination and challenge reveals 'masked' reactions to foods (see p. 98). Initially there may be a withdrawal reaction so that the symptoms worsen. A phase of hyperacute reactivity commonly follows and may last for weeks. After several weeks or months, tolerance to the previously reactive foods may follow.

Food re-challenge testing should therefore be timed to utilise the hyperacute phase for diagnosis. In this situation, symptom reactions are usually more severe and with a faster onset than those provoked by the same food in the same subject in the 'masked' state.

This post-elimination hyperacute phase, resulting in heightened speed and severity of symptom response, is not universally acknowledged. As a result, it has been suggested that non-immediate food hypersensitivity must be tested by prolonged challenges of up to 1 week per food. In most cases this is both time-consuming and unnecessary. Food tests can successfully be carried out at the rate of one or two foods per day providing that any symptoms from the preceding day's challenge are allowed to settle before the next test begins. Cereal grains are an exception, as they tend to produce delayed responses even in the unmasked state and should therefore be tested over 2 days.

Consider 5–10 day elimination of suspected missed reacting foods

It sometimes happens that, following a convincing response to the elimination diet, symptoms gradually return after a period of sequential food challenge without specific non-tolerated foods being identified. This may happen because symptom responses to a particular food have been overlooked. In this situation it is sometimes necessary to go back to a point in the sequential reintroduction prior to symptom recurrence and test each food again. In these circumstances, challenge

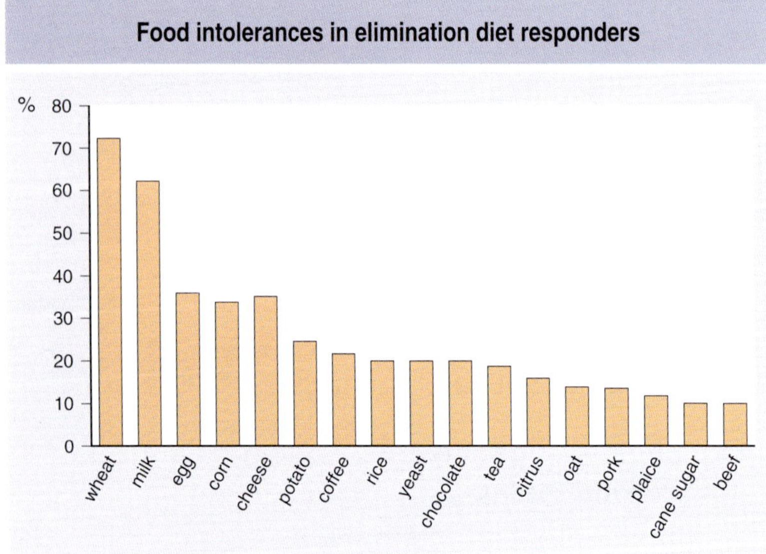

Fig 6.17 Food intolerances in elimination diet responders. Specific intolerances were identified by sequential food ingestion challenge. Data from: Radcliffe MJ. Clinical Methods for diagnosis. *Clin Immunol Allergy* 1982; **2**: 205-20.

with individual foods for periods of 5–10 days may be necessary.

Consider block challenge of foods untested so far

Food challenge testing should not usually continue for longer than 4 weeks, to avoid the possible development of tolerance. Provided that all frequently consumed and possibly implicated foods have been tested, and so long as the patient remains in remission, block challenge of the remaining foods can be considered.

Discount food intolerance

If the elimination regime was adequate and was followed conscientiously with proper attention to detail, then a negative conclusion can be drawn. Unfortunately, such standards are often difficult to achieve in practice, and inconclusive results are not uncommon. Great care must be taken in this situation to avoid leaving the patient with an inappropriately restricted diet that may be nutritionally or socially unacceptable.

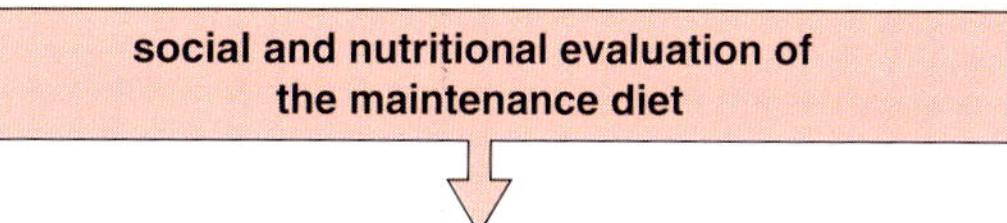

The involvement of a dietician with experience in the application and management of exclusion diets will be of considerable assistance throughout the whole food intolerance investigation. Once it is clear that significant improvement can be maintained by the avoidance of specific foods, the dietician is likely to be the best person to undertake an assessment of the nutritional, social, and psychological consequences of that diet (**Fig. 6.18**) In some cases the possibility of precipitating or exacerbating an eating disorder has to be borne in mind.

Social and nutritional evaluation of the maintenance diet

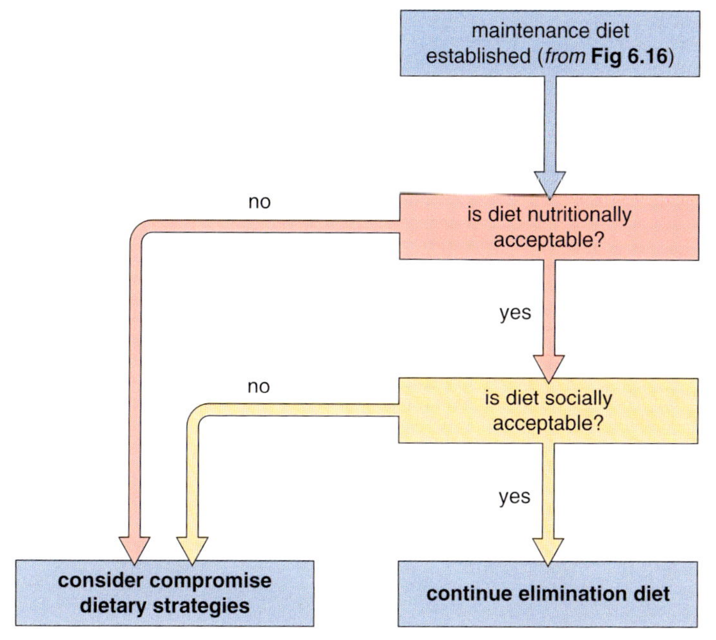

Fig 6.18 Social and nutritional evaluation of the maintenance diet is essential if the regime is to be successful.

Consider compromise dietary strategies

Where there are a number of non-tolerated foods, a compromise may be adopted. Those foods producing the most severe reaction are avoided, and those producing a less severe reaction may be eaten on a less frequent basis. In practice an interval of 3 days between exposures seems to be helpful in many cases. For the occasional patient who is greatly affected by many foods, a general regime of this type may be of great help. Such a diet is known as a *rotary diversified diet* (**Fig. 6.19**). Foods are divided into four groups of related foods and the diet is organized in such a way that no food is eaten more often than one day in four.

By this means the food-intolerant patient is able to maintain a wide food base and maintain nutritional adequacy. This is clearly to be preferred to a diet which is narrow and risks nutritional inadequacy. This kind of approach should, however, be reserved for the severely affected patient who cannot be helped in any other way.

Nutritional supplementation

Elimination diets can be associated with nutritional deficiency in some patients (e.g. in children, due to inappropriate enforcement of the diet by an over-zealous parent). However, nutritional improvements may occur in others. Indeed, benefits ascribed to specific food elimination may arise from improved intake of certain nutrients. Furthermore, apart from coeliac disease, in which the changes in the gut mucosa have been thoroughly investigated, there is little or no information available on the possible effect that regular ingestion of a non-tolerated food may have on absorption. For example, the bioavailability of ingested calcium might actually be improved by the exclusion of milk by a milk-intolerant patient. Dietary analysis by diary data or computer may be indicated in certain cases.

The social effects of elimination diets should not be underestimated. Most patients quickly learn that special diets attract a certain stigma, and for some this can be a considerable problem.

Disodium cromoglycate

Pre-ingestion of disodium cromoglycate (DSCG) has been shown to be protective against food allergy and intolerance in some patients, hindering both the development of immune complexes and the appearance of symptoms. Studies suggest that an IgE-mediated mechanism acts as a trigger to an alteration of mucosal permeability. It is possible that DSCG protects against symptoms by interfering with this process.

In practice it appears that symptoms precipitated by single-meal infringements to an established and effective elimination regime can be reduced or eliminated by adequate pre-treatment with DSCG. The contents of three capsules (300 mg) are tipped on the tongue, rinsed round the mouth with a little water half an hour before the meal. In some cases it may be possible to achieve a week or more of one-meal-a-day infringements without relapse, for example while on holiday. However, few sufferers find that DSCG continues to offer symptom protection when used for successive meals or prolonged periods.

Antihistamines

Antihistamines may be helpful in the management of urticaria, angioedema, rhinitis or the oral allergy syndrome, where these result from food allergy or intolerance. Pre-treatment with an antihistamine may reduce or prevent the effects of a single-meal infringement, and rapid post-treatment following inadvertent exposure may also be effective. Long-term antihistamine therapy is only indicated as part of the usual treatment for the resulting disorder (e.g. urticaria, rhinitis).

Continue the maintenance diet

The maintenance diet should be continued initially under the supervision of a dietician. Adverse responses to food may change with time, particularly in infancy, and so it is appropriate to reintroduce problem foods on a trial basis at intervals.

The four day rotary diversified diet

Day	Meat, poultry, and fish	Vegetables	Fruits	Beverages	Grains and flours	Nuts	Oils and fats	Sweetener
1	Beef Lamb	*Parsley family* Carrot, celery, parsnip, parsley *Fungi* Mushroom, yeast	*Rose family* Strawberry, raspberry *Apple family* Apple, pear	Milk Tea Apple juice	Oat	Brazil, cashew	Beef dripping Butter Cheese	Beet sugar
2	Fish Shellfish	*Sunflower family* Lettuce, chicory, endive, artichoke (Jer.) *Potato family* Tomato, peppers, potato	*Citrus family* Orange, lemon, grapefruit, lime *Avocado* *Rhubarb*	Orange juice, grapefruit juice (*citrus*) Chamomile tea *(sunflower family)*	Buckwheat, sunflower seed, tapioca	Filbert, hazel	Olive Sunflower oil Safflower oil	Maple syrup, maple sugar
3	Poultry Eggs	*Mustard family* Cabbage, brocolli, cauliflower, turnip *Gourd family* Marrow, cucumber, courgette	*Banana* *Melon* *Pineapple* *Gooseberry family* Gooseberry, currant	Pineapple juice Mint tea	Wheat Corn (maize) Rice	Walnut	Corn oil	Cane sugar Molasses
4	Pork Rabbit	*Sweet potato* *Legume family* Peas, beans, lentils, chick-pea, soya *Lily family* Onion, garlic, chive, asparagus, leek	*Grape family* Grape, raisin *Plum family* Cherry, peach, apricot *Palm family* Coconut, date	Grape juice Rosehip tea	Lentil Chick-pea Soya *(legumes)*	Peanut *(Legume)* Almond *(Plum)*	Peanut oil Soya oil	Date sugar Honey

Fig 6.19 The four day rotary diversified diet. Use unprocessed foods, fresh, frozen or dried. From Radcliffe MJ. *Clin Immunol Allergy* 1982; **2**: 205–20, with permission.

7 Eczema/Dermatitis

Rino Cerio

Introduction

Eczema and dermatitis are synonyms that refer to a polymorphic pattern of skin inflammation with characteristic clinical and pathological features. Clinical manifestations include itching, erythema, vesiculation, weeping and scaling, often complicated by secondary infection (**Fig. 7.1**). Histological features are a predominantly lympho-histiocytic infiltrate around upper dermal blood vessels, associated with epidermal spongiosis and varying degrees of acanthosis (**Fig. 7.2**).

Eczema/dermatitis accounts for an increasingly large proportion of all skin disorders. The eruption is a reaction to various stimuli, not all of which have been identified. Classification of the many clinical forms is difficult for the following reasons:

- The nomenclature is not universally agreed
- The condition may have multiple causes, and may be triggered by a range of external and internal factors, acting either alone or in combination
- Presentation may be acute, subacute or chronic
- It is not unusual for more than one form of dermatitis to affect the patient simultaneously.

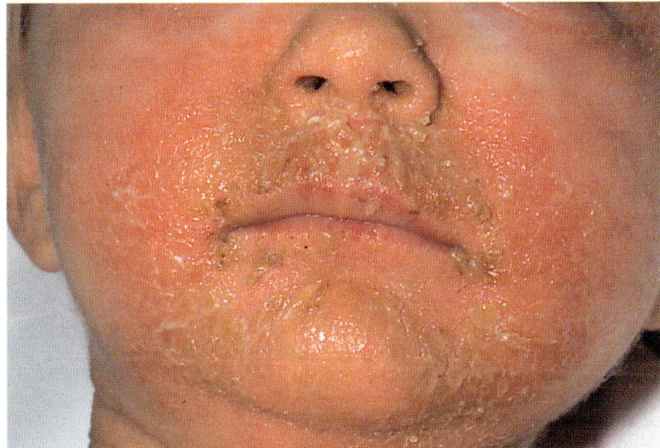

Fig. 7.1 Acute atopic eczema with impetiginization. Involvement of the face is common in infancy. In this child, secondary infection with *Staphylococcus aureus* required antibiotics in addition to topical corticosteroids.

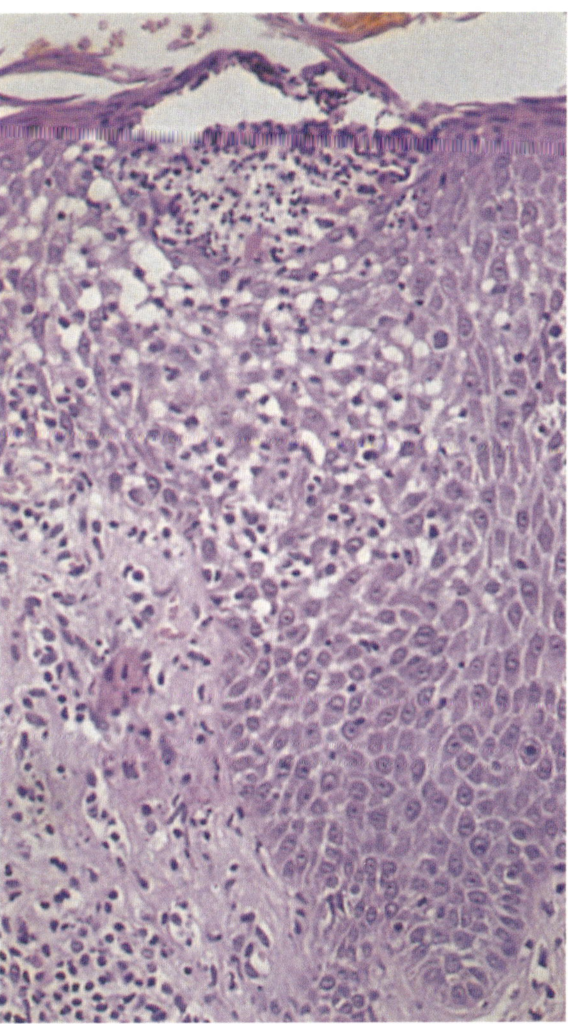

Fig. 7.2 Histopathology of eczema. This is a high-power view of the epidermis and papillary dermis in atopic eczema. There is epidermal thinning (acanthosis) and oedema (spongiosis), with a moderately heavy mononuclear cell infiltrate in the superficial dermis and epidermis (exocytosis). These features are seen in both exogenous and endogenous eczema; they are not specific to one subtype. The subcorneal pustule represents secondary impetiginization.

Exogenous eczema/dermatitis

Exogenous eczema/dermatitis is a common problem, accounting for up to 40% of all occupationally acquired illnesses, and up to 7% of all dermatological consultations. Exogenous eczema/dermatitis of the hands affects more than 2% of the population at some stage of their lives. In general, allergic dermatitis is less common than irritant dermatitis, but has a worse prognosis.

Endogenous eczema

Atopic eczema is the principle endogenous form. Atopy refers to a hereditary predisposition to produce IgE antibody. It predisposes the subject to diseases such as atopic eczema/dermatitis, asthma, conjunctivitis, and allergic rhinitis (*see* Chapter 1). Approximately 3–5% of infants below the age of 6 months are affected by atopic diseases. Sixty percent of patients with atopic eczema are affected by the age of one, rising to 80% in children aged 7 years. Recent studies have shown that although adulthood brings remission for some, 70% of those with severe dermatitis, and 60% with mild dermatitis, continue to suffer symptoms. Atopy is slightly more common in females.

Other endogenous forms are discussed below (*see* 'Diagnosis').

Unclassified eczema

A number of forms of eczema/dermatitis fall outside the endogenous/exogenous classification. They include asteatotic eczema, lichen striatus, lichen simplex chronicus, and drug-induced photodermatitis, and are discussed further below (*see* 'Diagnosis').

symptoms suggesting eczema/dermatitis

Patients with inflamed skin may complain of itching, redness and oozing. If the problem is acute then blisters may form with leaking fluid. A good guide to the severity of symptoms is to ask how the symptoms affect school, work and leisure time, and especially how they disturb sleep. Patients often do most scratching at night, and may complain of blood both on the skin and on bed linen. Secondary infection is common to most forms of eczema/dermatitis and is often described as weeping or 'wet' eczema (**Fig. 7.6**), as opposed to 'dry' scaly eczema (**Fig. 7.7**). Colour changes in the skin, as seen in pityriasis alba, reticulate pigmentation of the neck, and lichen simplex, may be due to either hypo- or hyperpigmentation. In cases of contact dermatitis the patient may already have identified the source of the problem (**Fig. 7.8**).

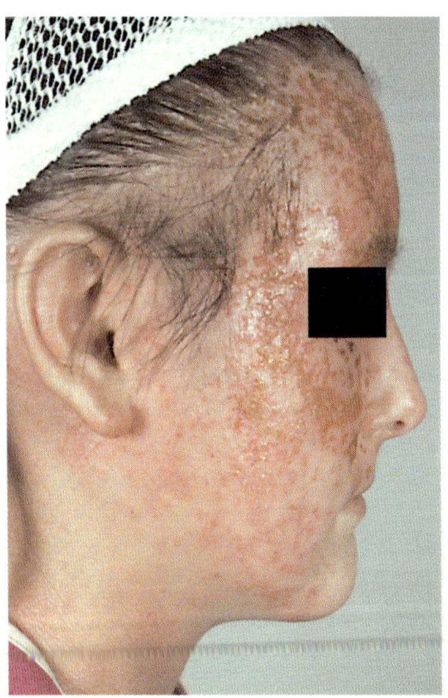

Fig. 7.6 'Wet' eczema This is usually patchy but widespread with yellow crusting and excoriations, without particular involvement of the flexures. This young atopic girl required hospital admission for intensive in-patient therapy.

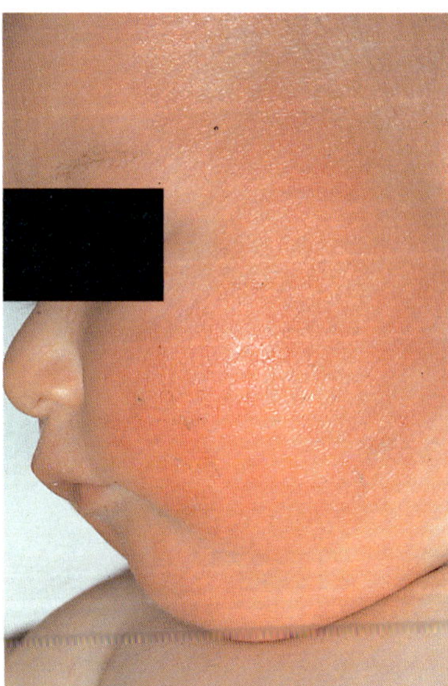

Fig. 7.7 'Dry' eczema. This starts with erythematous oedematous patches, followed by variable vesiculation and oozing. This baby has characteristic early distribution.

7 Eczema/Dermatitis

Rino Cerio

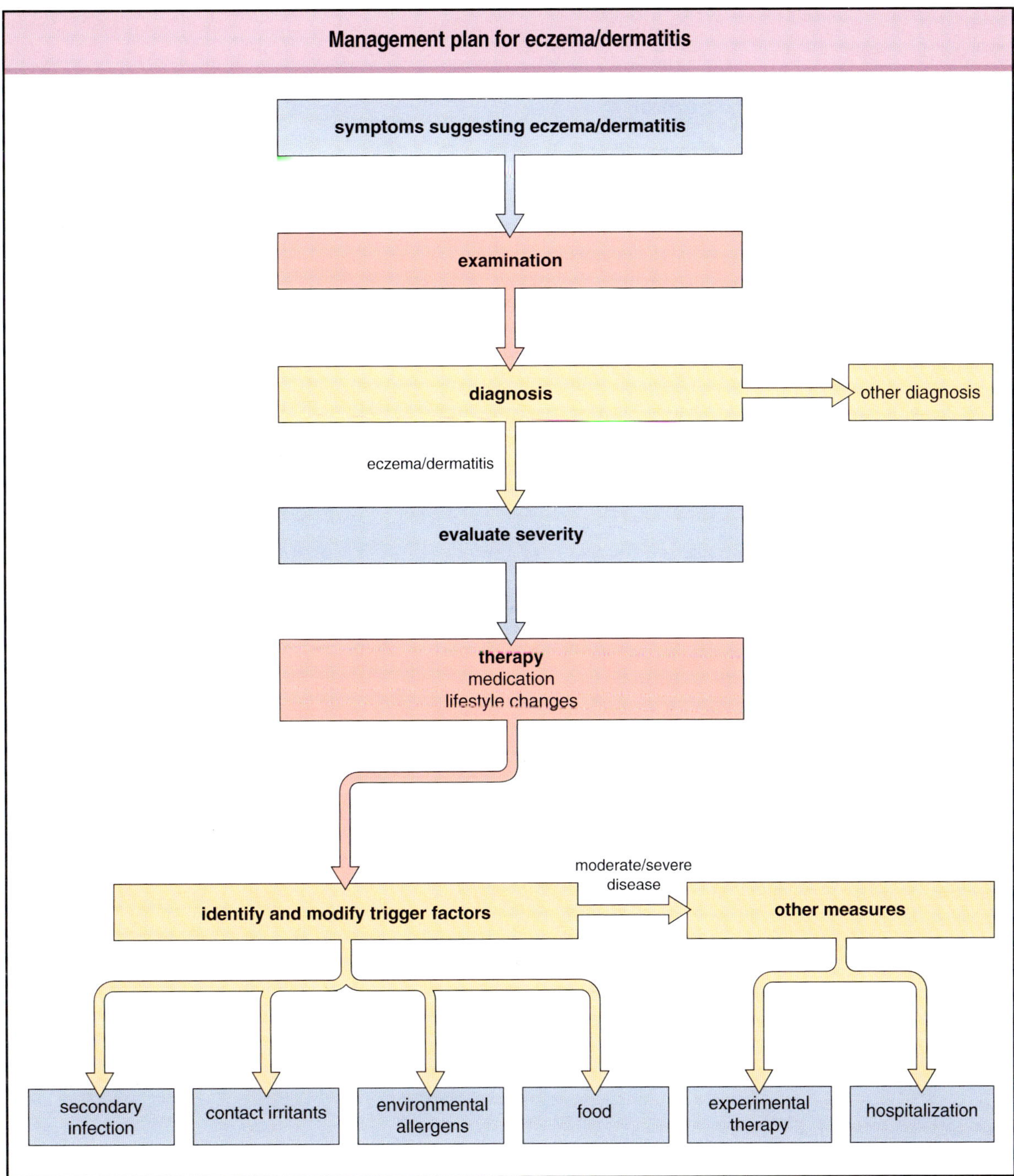

Eczema/dermatitis is usually classified as either *exogenous* or *endogenous* (**Fig. 7.3**). These two forms cannot be differentiated on the basis of histological appearance, or by immunological phenotyping of cell cytokines and adhesion molecules. Nevertheless, classification is important because it allows the investigator to identify contact allergies (which can be prevented by allergen avoidance), as well as certain treatable conditions that may also produce eczema-like skin lesions (**Figs 7.4 & 7.5**).

A classification of eczema/dermatitis	
Exogenous (contact)	Irritant (direct dose epidermal damage, non-allergic , e.g. with oils, abrasives, solvent, detergent) Allergic (type IV delayed hypersensitivity reaction) Phototoxic (photo-allergic and light aggravated) Immediate (type I hypersensitivity reaction)
Endogenous (constitutional)	Atopic Seborrhoeic Nummular (discoid) Pompholyx (dyshidrotic) Varicose/gravitational/stasis
Unclassified	Asteatotic Neurodermatitis/lichen simplex chronicus Nodular prurigo Lichen striatus

Fig. 7.3 A classification of eczema/dermatitis.

Conditions often confused with eczema
Fungal infections
Psoriasis
Scabies
Pityriasis rosea
Secondary syphilis
Drug reactions in photodermatitis
Erysipelas
Icthyosis
Acrodermatitis enteropathica
Histiocytosis X
X-linked agammaglobulinaemia

Fig. 7.4 Conditions often confused with eczema.

Some unusual causes of eczematous skin changes
Phenylketonuria
Wiskoff–Aldrich syndrome
Anhidrotic epidermal dysplasia
Pellagra
Malabsorption (essential fatty acids)

Fig. 7.5 Some unusual causes of eczematous skin changes.

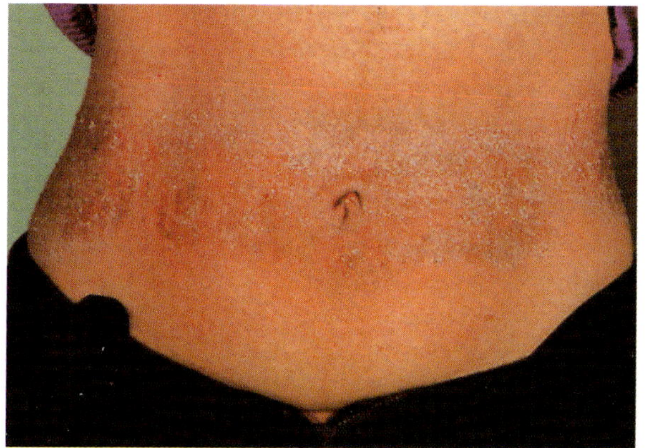

Fig. 7.8 Rubber contact allergy. This can sometimes be diagnosed by its distribution, as shown in this 30-year-old woman who became sensitive to the rubber in her underwear.

examination

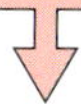

Management of eczema/dermatitis is based on accurate diagnosis and a full assessment of possible aetiological factors. Careful history taking and examination is therefore essential. Clinical findings depend on whether the eczema/dermatitis is acute, subacute or chronic. The patient's age and racial type influences the distribution (**Fig. 7.9**) and manifestation (**Figs 7.10 & 7.11**) of the rash.

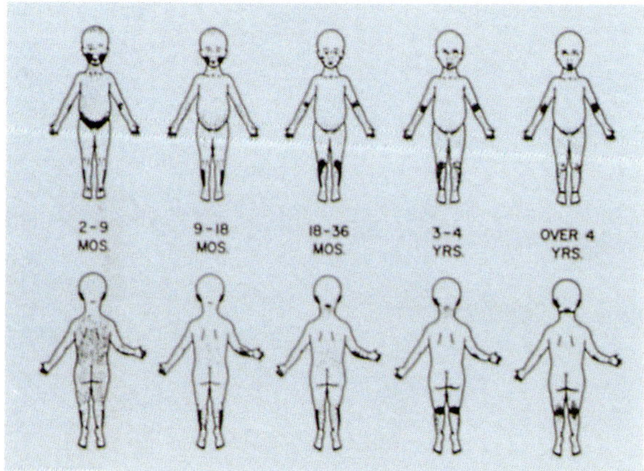

Fig. 7.9 The distribution of atopic eczema varies with age. Infantile eczema predominantly involves the cheeks and trunk, whereas from childhood onwards the eczema is mainly confined to the flexures.

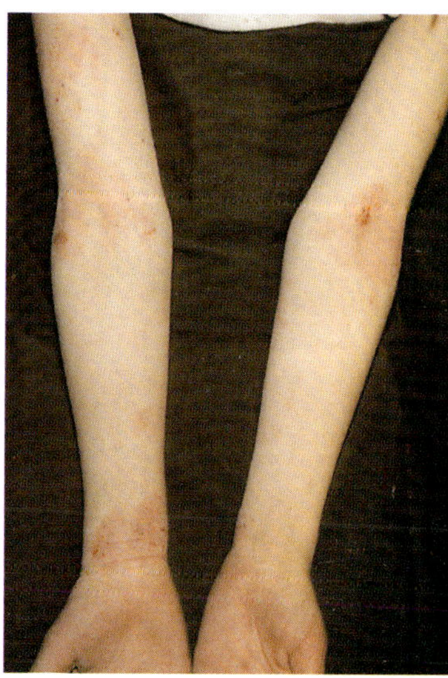

Fig 7.10 Atopic eczema classically occurs in the body flexures and is usually symmetrically distributed. In contrast to other allergic skin disorders, eczema affects the epidermis, and its appearance is modified by scratching and secondary infection.

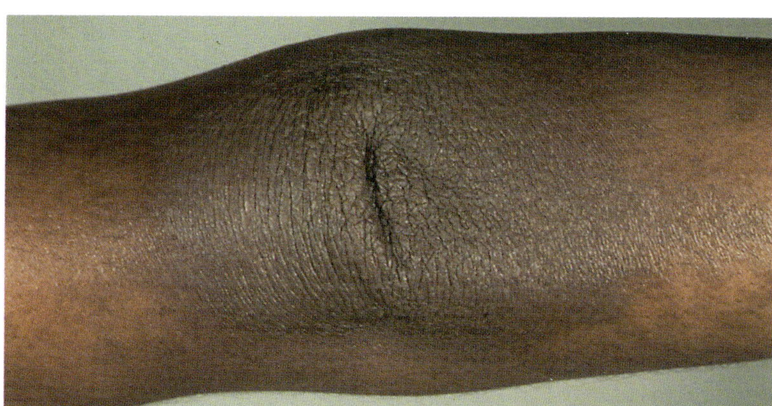

Fig. 7.11 Reverse pattern atopic eczema. In Afro-Caribbeans, atopic eczema tends to be more lichenified and papular, and it sometimes affects the extensor surfaces, rather than the flexures.

Atopic individuals may have associated conditions, such as allergic rhinitis, allergic conjunctivitis and asthma. Identification of associated physical signs, such as dry skin, Dennie–Morgan infra-orbital folds (*see* **Fig. 1.15**), keratosis pilaris (**Fig. 7.12**), ichthyosis vulgaris, pityriasis alba (**Fig. 7.13**) and juvenile plantar dermatosis (**Fig. 7.14**), may help establish an atopic diathesis.

Secondary complications, such as bacterial (**Fig. 7.15**) or viral (**Figs 7.16 & 7.17**) infection, may be present.

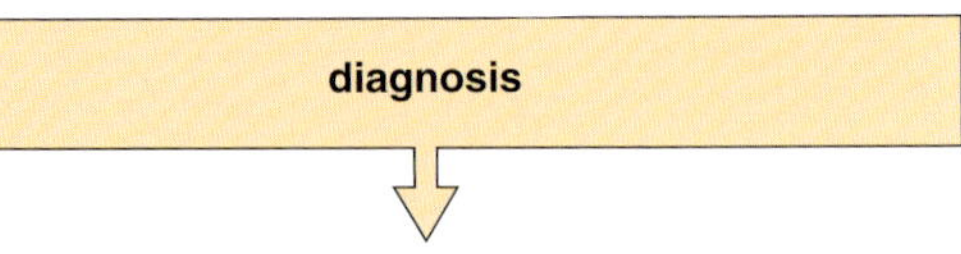

A full examination and history should make it possible either to diagnose a form of eczema/dermatitis, or to establish an alternative diagnosis.

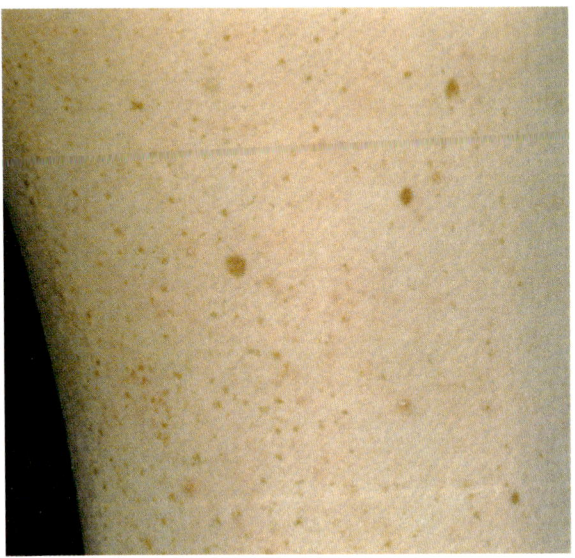

Fig. 7.12 Keratosis pilaris. This condition is a relatively common autosomal dominant disorder due to hyperkeratosis of the hair follicles, which become filled with horny plugs. The changes begin in childhood and improve with age. They are usually confined to the outer aspects of the arms and thighs and rarely involve the face. Association with atopy is recognized.

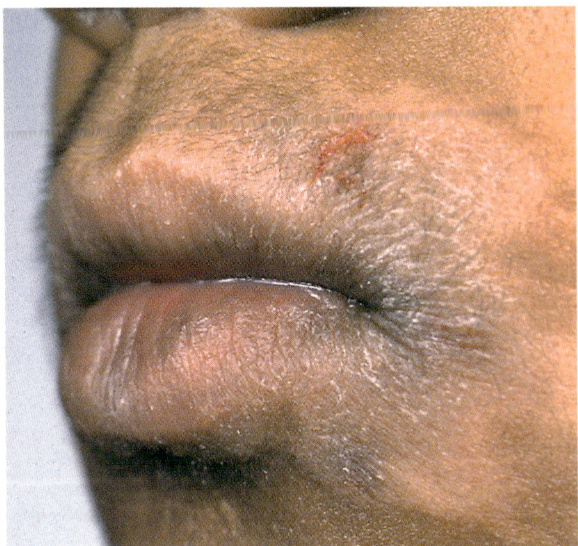

Fig. 7.13 Pityriasis alba. This is characterized by hypopigmented scaly patches in the perioral region, on the cheeks and sometimes on the proximal limbs. It is found in otherwise normal patients and in those with atopic eczema. It invariably resolves with age.

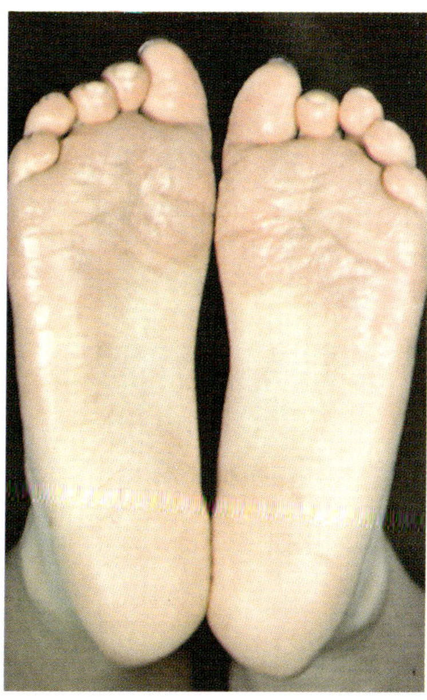

Fig. 7.14 Juvenile plantar dermatosis. Some feel this condition is a manifestation of atopy. The skin of the weight-bearing areas of the feet becomes dry and shiny, with deep painful fissures. Trainer shoes, which are popular among children, often cause excessive sweating and may be the true culprit.

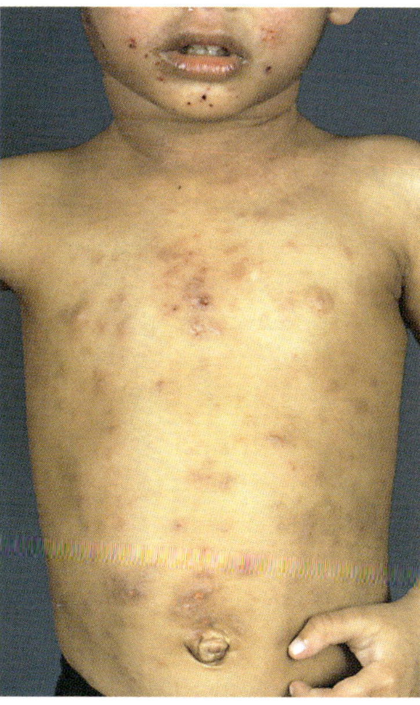

Fig. 7.15 Widespread excoriation and crusting. This often indicates secondary bacterial infection which, by release of exotoxin, aggravates atopic eczema.

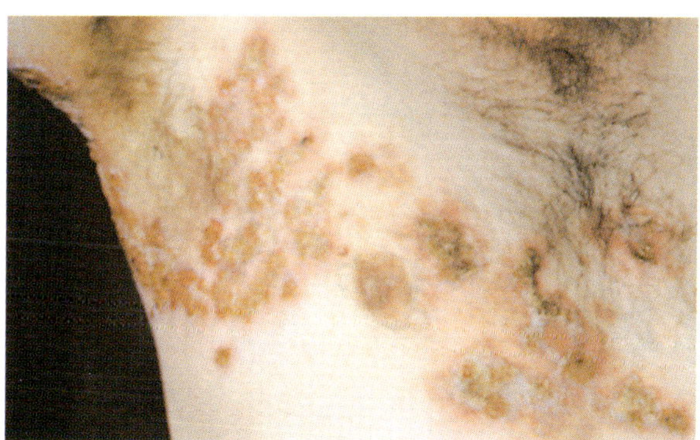

Fig. 7.16 Herpes zoster in eczema. This young man with atopic eczema developed shingles of the T4 dermatome. The eruption became secondarily infected with *Staphylococcus aureus* (impetiginized). Patients with atopic eczema are more susceptible to skin infections.

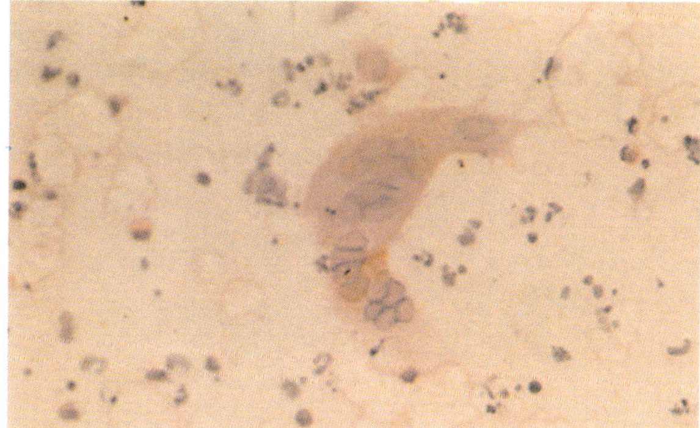

Fig. 7.17 Herpes infection. A Tzanck test is useful in confirming a herpetic infection, whether simplex or zoster. This is performed by removing the roof of a fresh vesicle, scraping the base and examining the cells microscopically. The cells here are multinucleated, which is typical of this viral infection.

Exogenous eczema/dermatitis

Exogenous or contact dermatitis is a likely diagnosis if:

- The inflammation has followed contact with known irritants or allergens (**Fig. 7.18**)
- The eruption clears when the patient is on holiday or off work
- The eruption is asymmetrical and has a linear/rectilinear configuration (pattern recognition is important)
- The patient is atopic (irritants especially) (*see* Chapter 1).

Endogenous eczema/dermatitis

Atopic eczema

Clinical presentation of atopic eczema varies depending on the age and race of the patient (*see* **Figs 7.10 & 7.11**). Trigger factors are listed in **Fig. 7.19**.

Some common allergens in contact dermatitis

Allergen	Sources
Nickel	Jewellery, jean studs, bra clips, tools
Balsam of Peru	Perfumes, citrus fruits
Dichromate	Cement, leather, matches
Paraphenylenediamine	Hair dyes, clothing
Rubber chemicals	Shoes, clothing, gloves
Colophony (rosin)	Sticking plaster, collodium
Neomycin	Topical medicaments
Benzocaine	Topical anaesthetics
Parabens	Preservatives in cosmetics and creams
Wood alcohols	Lanolin, cosmetics, creams
Imidazolidinyl urea	Preservative in creams and cosmetics
Formaldehyde (acqueous)	Clothing, cosmetics, glues, paper
Epoxy resin	Glues

Fig. 7.18 Some common allergens in contact dermatitis.

Trigger factors in atopic eczema

Irritants	Detergents, clothing, sweat
Allergens	Food, especially intolerance in infants (aged up to 18 months) to cows' milk and hens' eggs
Infection	*Staphylococcus aureus* via superantigen exotoxins Viral, such as HPV, molluscum contagiosum and widespread herpes and vaccinia (eczema herpeticum)
Stress	Often coincides with exacerbations, especially in teenagers and adults

Fig. 7.19 Trigger factors in atopic eczema.

Seborrhoeic eczema/dermatitis

This is usually confined to areas rich in sebum. Perifollicular, erythematous, pink or yellow scaly lesions develop on the face and scalp (**Fig. 7.20**). The combination of sebum, hyperhidrosis and overgrowth of *Pityrosporum ovale* produces inflammation. In newborns, seborrhoeic eczema/dermatitis presents as cradle cap (**Fig. 7.21**).

Nummular or discoid eczema/dermatitis

This is a localized, coin-shaped, acute inflammation occurring on limbs, and is often seen with secondary infection (**Fig. 7.22**). It is common in middle-aged men with a personal or family history of atopy. In its exudative form it is also known as neurodermatitis, while its dry form is known as lichen simplex (**Fig. 7.23**). Another, even

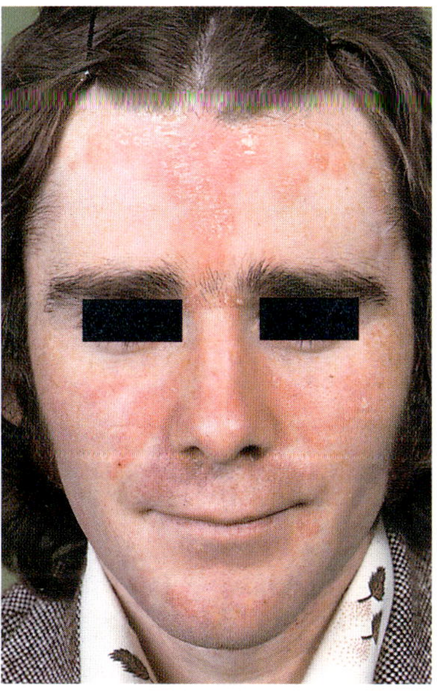

Fig. 7.20 In adults, seborrhoeic dermatitis is found chiefly in young men. The face is commonly affected. This condition is not related to infantile seborrheic dermatitis.

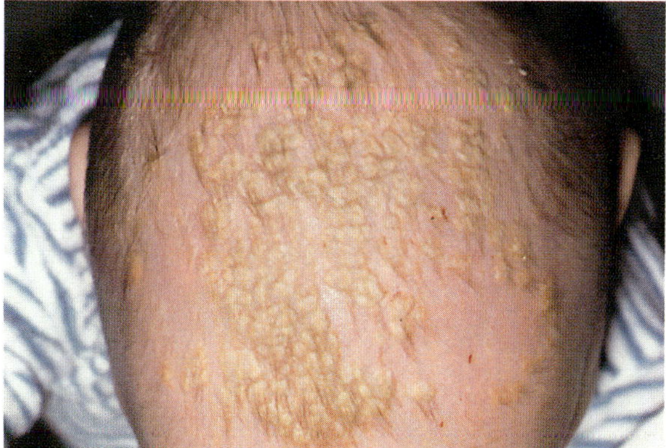

Fig. 7.21 Infantile seborrhoeic dermatitis. This often affects the scalp, presenting with red and yellow adherent scales. Despite the florid eruption, which can be widespread, and in contrast to atopic eczema, the infant is relatively asymptomatic. The condition is self-limiting.

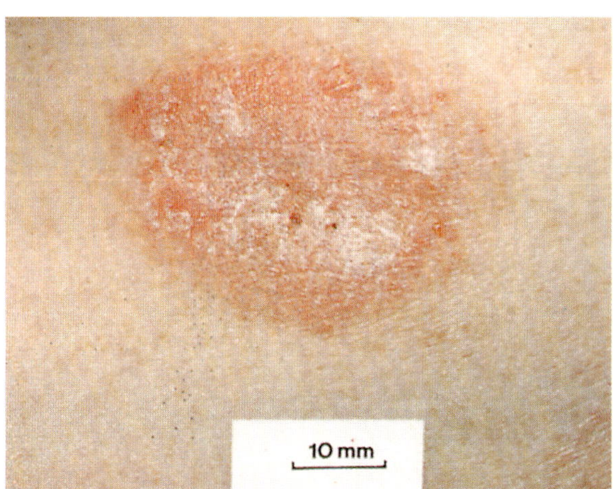

Fig. 7.22 Nummular or discoid eczema in a 39-year-old man. The lesions are subcute, with erythema, mild oedema and some vesiculation.

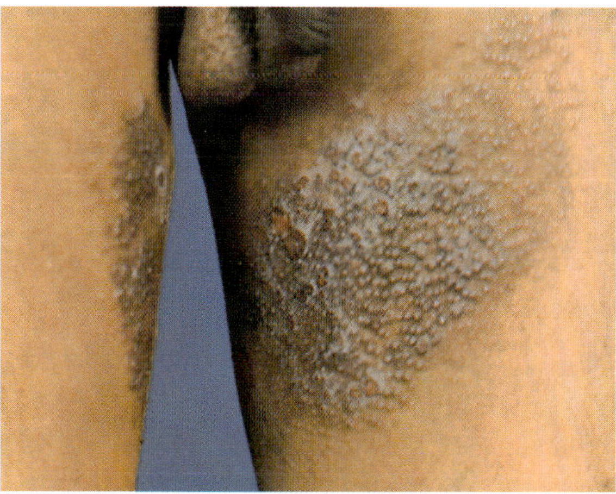

Fig. 7.23 Lichenified atopic eczema. Prolonged scratching and rubbing can lead to severe hyperpigmentation and lichenification. If localized, the condition is known as lichen simplex.

more localized form of lichenification is nodular prurigo (**Fig. 7.24**).

Pompholyx/dyshidrotic eczema/dermatitis
This is one of the most unpleasant acute and recurrent forms of eczema, with epidermal oedema (spongiosis) leading to vesicles and even bullae. It affects the extremities in young adults, and starts on the lateral aspects of fingers (**Fig. 7.25**). It is provoked by heat, stress, or an active fungal infection of the feet (an id reaction). Rarely, in highly sensitized individuals, it is triggered by ingested nickel. Secondary infection is common.

Varicose, gravitational or statis eczema
This is a chronic condition affecting the lower medial aspect of the leg in older adults. It is accompanied by venous insufficiency, varicose veins, oedema, haemosiderin deposition and lipodermatosclerosis (**Fig. 7.26**). If poorly

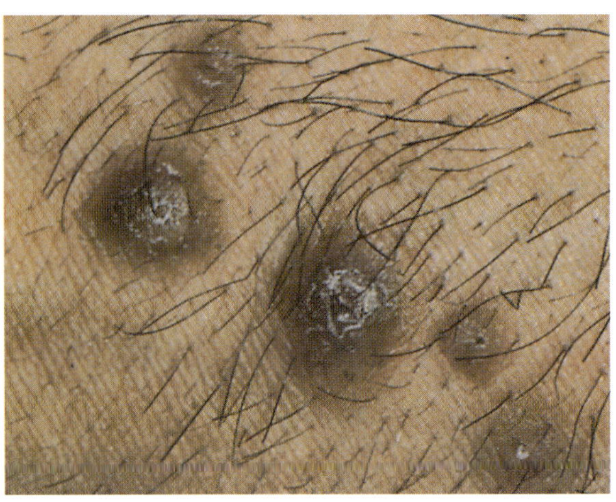

Fig. 7.24 Nodular prurigo. This condition usually affects middle-aged and elderly females, who present with pruritic nodules on the legs and arms. A few cases may have an underlying iron deficiency, but the majority are a form of neurodermatitis.

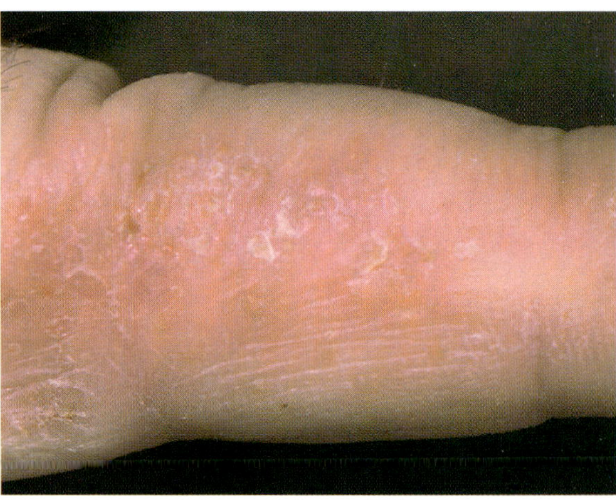

Fig. 7.25 Pompholyx. This young man developed pruritic vesicles on the lateral aspects of many of his fingers, especially when he was under stress. The eruption resolved with regular use of emollients and topical corticosteroids, sometimes used under occlusion.

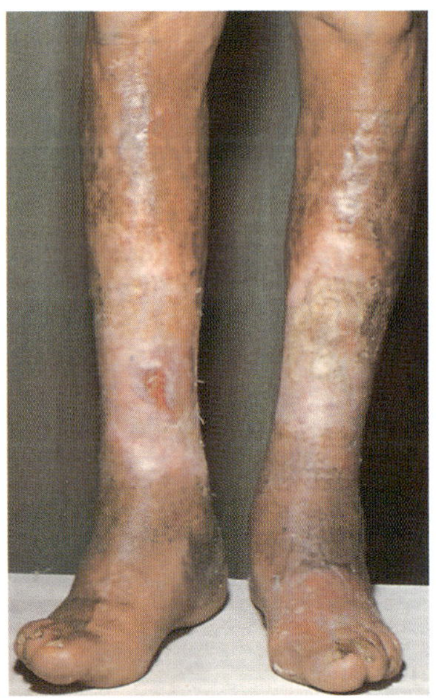

Fig. 7.26 Stasis eczema. This is commonly seen in elderly females, in association with venous insufficiency or frank ulceration. This 68-year-old woman's legs also show marked pigmentation due to haemosiderin deposition.

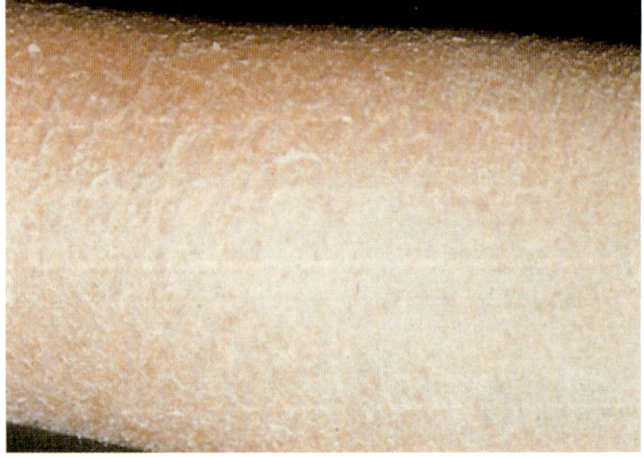

Fig. 7.27 Asteatotic eczema (eczema crequalé). This is a common form of endogenous eczema affecting the elderly. The characteristic fissuring of the skin gives a 'crazy paving' appearance. Often it is well controlled by avoidance of irritants and the regular use of topical emollients.

Medication

Corticosteroids

Corticosteroids are effective when used topically. As a rule, the least potent effective agent should be used. The dose should be titrated to avoid long-term side-effects during maintenance therapy (**Fig. 7.38**).

The choice of drug varies according to the patient's age, and the extent and location of the lesions. The recently developed, highly specific, once-daily topical corticosteroids, such as mometasone furoate, have been shown to be highly effective with minimal adverse effects, even in children (**Fig. 7.39**).

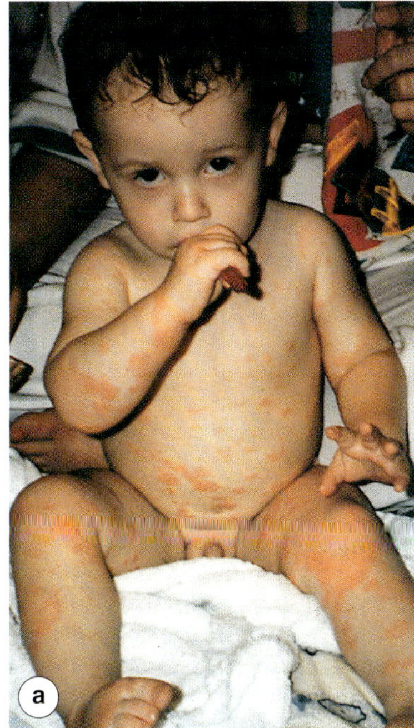

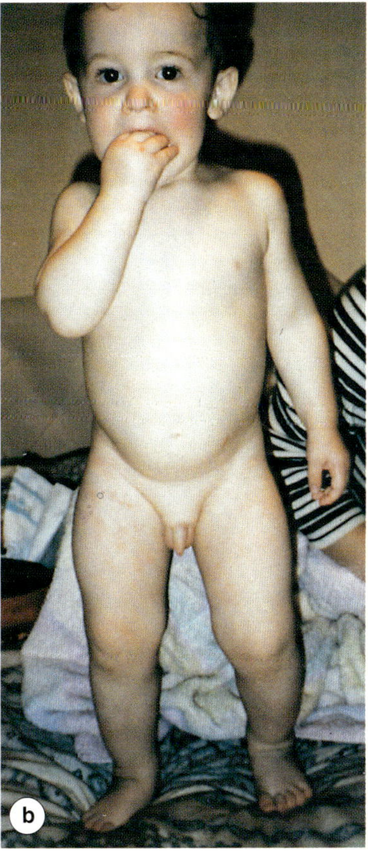

Fig. 7.39 Infantile eczema before and after a short course of once-daily treatment with a topical corticosteroid (mometasone furoate). This infant had developed atopic eczema shortly after receiving mumps/measles/rubella (MMR) immunization.

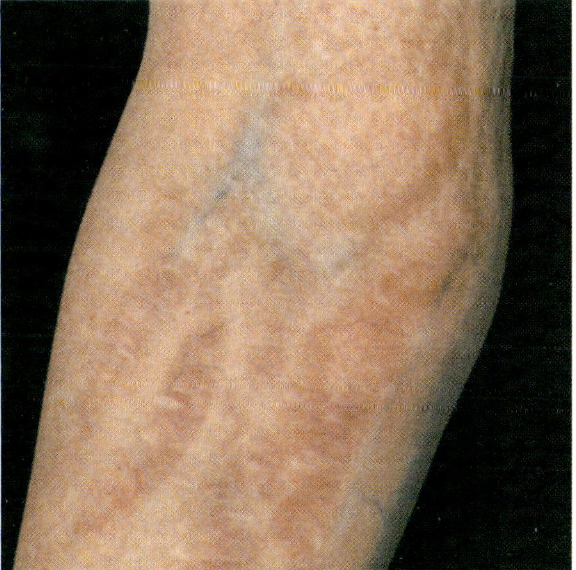

Fig. 7.38 Corticosteroid-induced striae. These permanent striae in a patient with atopic eczema were caused by over-use of potent topical corticosteroid therapy. It is essential to avoid the inappropriate and/or excessive use of corticosteroids in such treatment for all dermatological conditions. Additional complications of excessive corticosteroid therapy include delayed healing of wounds, masking of fungal and bacterial infections, and exacerbation of pustular acne.

Guide to required amounts of topical corticosteroids		
	4 year old	**70kg adult**
Trunk (front/back)	40gm	120gm
All four limbs	70gm	180gm
Whole body	120gm	340gm

Fig. 7.40 Guide to required amounts of topical corticosteroids. The amounts shown are those necessary for twice-daily treatment for 14 days.

Fingertip units guide for application of corticosteroids	
Trunk (front/back)	8 FTU daily
Legs and arms	12 FTU daily
Whole body (includes hands/feet)	24 FTU daily

Fig. 7.41 Fingertip units guide for application of corticosteroids. A fingertip unit is defined as the quantity of corticosteroid reaching from the fingertip to the distal interpharyngeal joint.

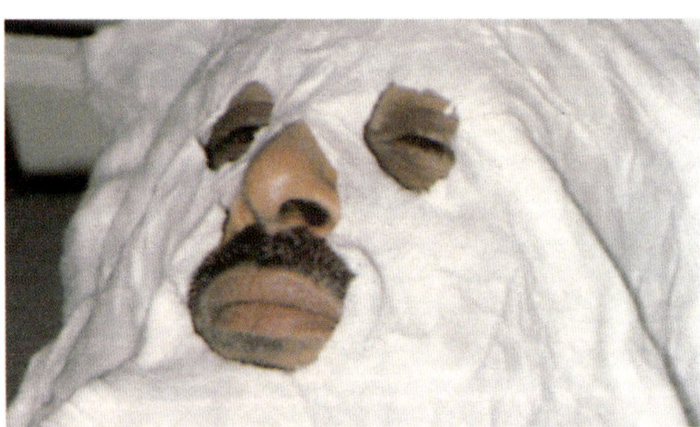

Fig. 7.42 'Wet wrap' therapy. This old-fashioned but simple technique is very effective in re-hydrating the skin, and it may be valuable in severe, dry, flaking eczema/dermatitis. The technique also provides considerable symptomatic relief, especially where pruritus is a major problem. If a large part of the body is to be treated in this way, care should be taken to avoid inducing hypothermia as a result of evaporation from the wrap.

Patients and doctors must ensure that an adequate supply of corticosteroid is maintained (**Fig. 7.40**). 'Fingertip units' can help patients and parents to use the correct amount of topical steroid at each application (**Fig. 7.41**). Regular, correct application of topical agents is important. They must not be used at the same time as moisturisers, as this will dilute their effect.

For severe cases, 'wet wrap' occlusive therapy, with or without steroids, can be of great benefit (**Fig. 7.42**). Alternatively, localized lichenified patches may require corticosteroid under occlusion to enhance penetration of the thickened skin.

Systemic steroid treatment should be reserved for very severe cases. Although symptom relief can be dramatic, withdrawal of the treatment often produces a rebound flare. Systemic steroids used chronically are associated with serious side-effects.

Anti-pruritic agents

Other potentially beneficial topical agents include urea as a hydrating agent, zinc oxide for healing, and coal tar for lichenified inflamed skin. Most can be used singly or in combination in impregnated occlusive bandages. They also have the benefit of protecting the skin from external trauma.

The newer antihistamines (H_1) such as loratadine can help many patients with intense pruritis, although the older sedative agents probably work centrally by sedation, with little direct effect demons-trated to date. Tachyphylaxis is also recognized with the older drugs.

Lifestyle changes

Education and self-management is crucial to both short- and long-term improvement, so patients must be provided all necessary information on their condition. For example, the dry, sensitive skin of affected patients is easily irritated by soaps, solvents and fabrics, such as wool and nylon, so patients should modify their lifestyle and surroundings accordingly. Fingernails should be kept short to minimize the risk of exacerbations due to scratching

In moderate/severe cases, support from dermatology paediatric nurse specialists is invaluable to ensure compliance. A home visit by the doctor or nurse may aid the assessment of the eczema, helping to identify underlying causes and the most appropriate management. In some countries, 'parent schools' have shown to be particularly successful in encouraging a self-management philosophy, especially for families with an atopic child. Support self-help groups, both local and national, offer a similar service.

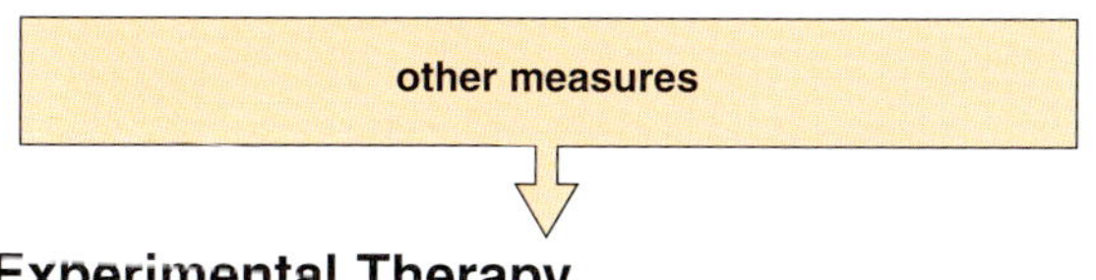

Experimental Therapy

Modulation of the immune response occurs with both *photochemotherapy (PUVA)* and *UVB irradiation*. Some light responsive eczema can benefit from this but treatment is long term and requires a well-motivated patient.

Oral evening primrose oil (linoleic and gamma linoleic acid) has been shown to have a beneficial effect in some patients, often with mild disease.

Steroid-sparing systemic agents, such as *cyclosporin*, may have a dramatic clinical effect, although relapses occur on discontinuation of the drug. Moreover, the drug is associated with serious side-effects, such as renal impairment, and with a long-term risk of lymphoma. In elderly patients, *azothiaprine* may be a better alternative, but is also associated with a risk of serious bone marrow and carcinogenic side-effects. *Dapsone* has been used in a similar way, with mixed benefit.

Thymopentin is a polypeptide that mimics thymopoietin, a thymic hormone affecting T lymphocytes. Studies have shown limited improvement after 6 weeks, with a high relapse rate.

Positive results with atopic eczema have also been shown with *traditional Chinese herbal mixtures*, but only in some patients with 'dry' eczema. The possibility of hepatotoxicity must be carefully monitored if such mixtures are used.

Patients with atopic dermatitis may improve with regular subcutaneous injections of *recombinant interferon-gamma*, but side-effects and relapse are seen once the treatment is discontinued.

New anti-inflammatory and immunomodulatory agents are likely to be developed as the pathogenesis of eczema/dermatitis is elucidated.

Hospitalization

If outpatient treatment fails then more regular day care treatment or even hospitalization nearly always helps to restore confidence and ensure compliance. It also educates patients and parents about long-term measures to deal with the problem.

identify and modify trigger factors

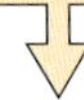

Secondary infection

Secondary infection is important in both acute and chronic forms of eczema. Patients and carers need to be aware of the importance of treating these complications. Infected exacerbations require a combination of antiseptic, topical antibiotic, and systemic antibiotic for bacterial infection, and topical and/or systemic antiviral treatment for herpes. Secondary infections with herpes may require urgent hospital admission and isolation (**Fig. 7.43**). Some patients with severe involvement may require long-term anti-infection measures.

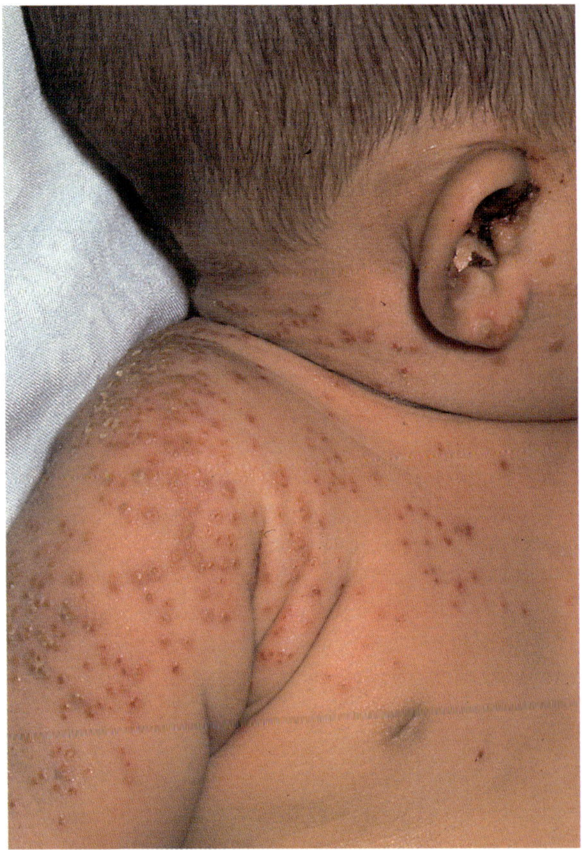

Fig. 7.43 Eczema herpeticum (Kaposi's varicelliform eruption). In this infant, herpes simplex spread to cause severe vesicular necrotic lesions requiring emergency in-patient treatment. This complication can also occur following chickenpox.

Contact irritants

Contact allergy patch testing should be carried out, and repeated at intervals if an offending agent is suspected. The recently recognized contact allergies to topical steroid molecules present a difficult problem, and require investigation and exclusion. Irritants must be avoided in all affected patients with all forms of eczema/dermatitis, as the avoidance of contact allergens can be curative.

Environmental allergens

The role of specific environmental allergens can sometimes be confirmed by skin prick test or radioallergosorbent test (RAST) IgE measurements. However, avoidance of allergens is often difficult, and may not even be beneficial.

Food

Except for atopic infants, specific food avoidance is not often beneficial. Intolerance to cows' milk and hens' eggs is most common in infancy, so milk substitutes and delayed weaning is recommended advice for some severely affected youngsters.

Provoking factors may be exogenous or endogenous (**Fig. 8.5**). As well as histamine, many mediators can result in symptoms and signs of urticaria including prostaglandins, leukotrienes, platelet activating factors, kallikrein, kinin system neuropeptides, and cytokines (**Fig. 8.6**).

Provoking factors in urticaria
Exogenous factors
Food and food additives (e.g. shellfish, tartrazine)
Drugs (topical and systemic)
Insect bites
Pollen
Inhalants
Animal dander
Physical stimuli
Endogenous factors
Intestinal parasites
Connective tissue disorder, e.g. systemic lupus erythematosus
Autoimmune thyroid disease
Diabetes
Carcinoma/lymphoma
Pregnancy

Fig. 8.5 Provoking factors in urticaria.

Although Type I allergy is an important cause of urticaria, but non-allergic mechanisms are more common. Non-allergic urticaria or angioedema may occur on first exposure to a provoking substance or event, whereas IgE-mediated urticaria requires sensitization from prior exposure to the provoking agent or a related substance.

Types of Urticaria

IgE-dependent urticaria

This is due to a Type I hypersensitivity reaction mediated by IgE (and sometimes IgG4). Allergens may be encountered by ingestion (of food), by inhalation, by injection, from parasites, from infections, or from insect bites.

Chronic idiopathic urticaria

About three quarters of patients who present with urticaria have the chronic idiopathic form. The majority of these patients are not atopic, and have normal IgE concentrations. Chronic idiopathic urticaria affects middle-aged women in particular, and recent studies have shown that an IgG anti-Ig autoantibody can be identified in a proportion of these cases.

The onset is usually fairly abrupt and no precipitating causes are apparent. Most cases resolve spontaneously within two years, but symptoms may persist for 10 years or more in about 20% of patients. Abnormalities of complement factors have been demonstrated in some patients, mainly in so-called urticarial vasculitis.

Physical urticaria

A large number of variants of urticaria provoked by physical stimuli have been described. Their major characteristics are summarized in **Fig. 8.7**.

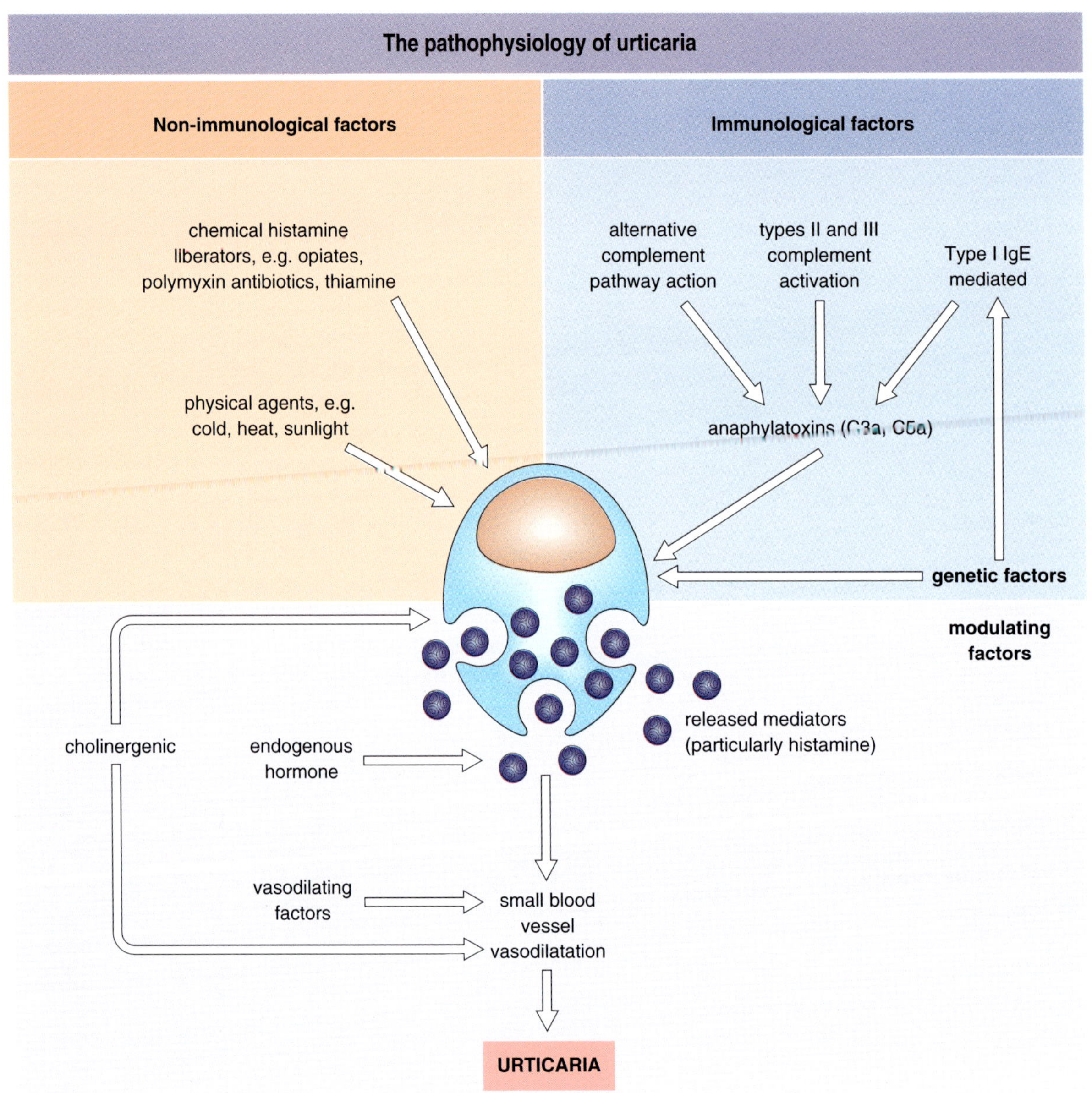

Fig. 8.6 The pathophysiology of urticaria. Mast cells can be stimulated to release mediators by various immunological and non-immunological factors. Histamine is often the mediator responsible for the cutaneous vascular changes seen in urticaria, but many other naturally occurring substances may be involved. IgE antibodies are often, but not always, involved in mast cell degranulation.

Types of physical urticaria									
Urticaria	**Relative frequency**	**Precipitant**	**Time of onset**	**Duration**	**Local symptoms**	**Systemic symptoms**	**Tests**	**Mechanism**	**Treatment**
Symptomatic dermographism	Most frequent	Stroking skin	Minutes	2–3 hours	Irregular, pruritic weals	None	Scratch skin	Possible role of adenosine triphosphate; substance P; possible direct pharmacological mechanism	Continuous antihistamine regimen; combined H_1 and H_2 blockers
Delayed pressure urticaria	Frequent	Pressure	3–12 hrs	8–24 hrs	Diffuse tender swelling	Flu-like symptoms	Apply weight	Unknown	Avoidance of precipitants; if severe, antihistamines or low doses of corticosteroids given for systemic effect
Solar urticaria	Uncommon	Various wavelengths of light	2–5 minutes	15 mins to 3 hours	Pruritic weals	Wheezing; dizziness; syncope	Photo test	Passive transfer; reverse passive transfer; IgE; possibly histamine	Avoidance of precipitants; antihistamines; sunscreens; chloroquine phosphate regimen for short time
Cold urticaria	Frequent	Cold	2–5 minutes	1–2 hours	Pruritic weals	Wheezing; syncope; drowning	Apply ice-filled copper beaker to arm, immerse in cold water	Passive transfer; reverse passive transfer; IgE (IgM); histamine vasculitis can be induced	Antihistamines; desensitization; avoidance of precipitants
Heat urticaria	Rare	Heat	2–5 minutes, rarely delayed	1 hour	Pruritic weals	None	Apply hot water-filled cylinder to arm	Possibly histamine; possibly complement	Antihistamines; desensitization; avoidance of precipitants
Cholinergic urticaria	Very frequent	General over-heating of body, exercise, stress	2–20 minutes	30 mins to 1 hour	Papular, pruritic weals	Syncope; diarrhoea; vomiting; salivation; headaches	Baths in hot water, exercise until perspiring, inject methacholine chloride	Passive transfer; possibly immunoglobulin; product of sweat gland stimulation; histamine; reduced protease inhibitor	Application of cold water or ice to skin; antihistamines; refractory period; anticholinergics
Aquagenic urticaria	Rare	Water contact	Several minutes to 30 minutes	30–45 minutes	Papular, pruritic weals	None reported	Apply water compresses to skin	Unknown	Avoidance of precipitants; antihistamines; application of inert oil
Vibratory angioedema	Very rare	Vibrating against skin	2–5 mins	1 hour	Angio-edema	None reported	Apply body of vibrating mixer to forearm	Unknown	Avoidance of precipitants

Fig. 8.7 Types of physical urticaria. Modified from: Jarizza JL and Smith EB. *Arch Dermatol* 1982; **118**: 198.

Dermographism

In this common form of urticaria (**Fig. 8.8**), mast cells in the skin release histamine after rubbing or scratching. The linear weals are therefore an exaggerated weal and flare reaction, which can be elicited as a physical sign.

Delayed pressure urticaria

As the name suggests, this type of urticaria develops after 3–6 hours and can last 48 hours. It occurs particularly on the feet, hands and buttocks, and is probably mediated by kinins and prostaglandins, rather than by histamine.

Temperature-dependent urticaria

These types of urticaria can be produced in the clinic by exposing the skin to extremes of temperature. Urticaria may be provoked by heat or by cold (**Fig. 8.9**). Occasionally, cold urticaria is the presenting feature of cryoglobulinaemia.

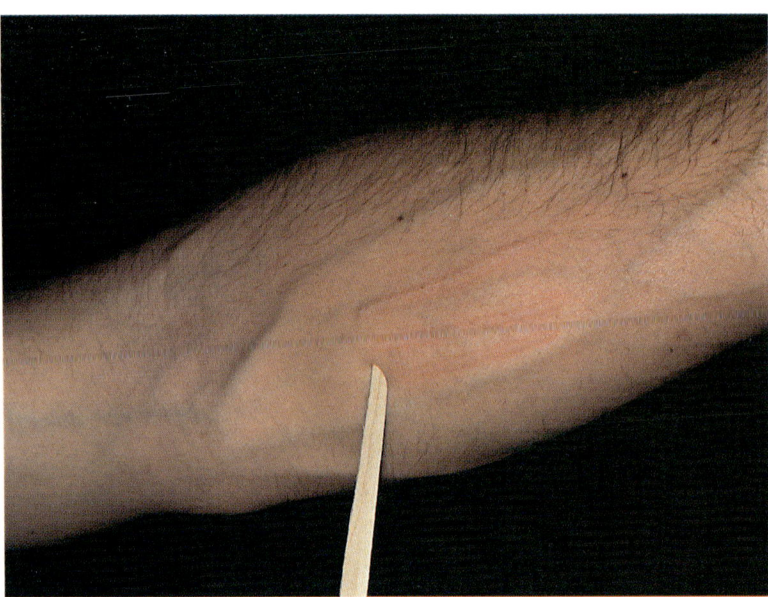

Fig. 8.8 Dermographism is the most common form of physical urticaria. It may be hereditary or acquired. A linear weal and flare reaction develops within 2–3 minutes of scratching normal skin with a blunt instrument or finger. Antihistamine treatment is usually effective and undue trauma to the skin should be avoided.

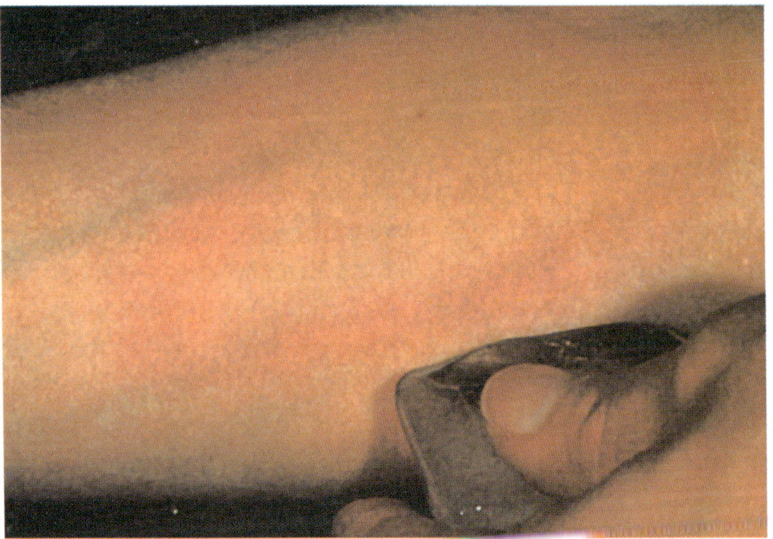

Fig. 8.9 Cold urticaria developed in this patient within minutes of holding an ice cube against the skin; it lasted for several hours. The condition may be inherited as an autosomal dominant trait, but it is usually acquired, and there is no obvious reason for its onset. In severe cases, similar reactions may be provoked by cold air or water, and there may be oropharyngeal oedema on the ingestion of cold liquids. In very sensitive patients, reactions resembling anaphylactic shock may occur. Antihistamine treatment may be helpful.

Solar urticaria

This form of urticaria may be IgE-mediated, but some patients with solar urticaria have erythropoietic protoporphyria.

Cholinergic urticaria

Strenuous exercise, anxiety, or occasionally heat, are all capable of eliciting this disorder. The eruption tends to be more papular than is the case with idiopathic urticaria (**Fig. 8.10**). It is mediated by acetylocholine, which is released from parasympathetic nerves in the skin and causes vasodilatation.

Fig. 8.10 Cholinergic urticaria is a distinctive type of urticaria in which small pruritic papules develop after stimuli such as exercise, stress and heat (e.g. taking a hot bath). The condition usually affects young adults, and appears on the upper trunk, but it may be more widespread. The lesions are characteristically very small and the episodes are short-lived, lasting 15–30 minutes. Itching is prominent and systemic symptoms, such as wheezing, rarely occur. Treatment with antihistamines may be helpful, and hydroxyzine hydrochloride – which also has a minor sedative action – may be particularly beneficial.

Contact urticaria

This type of urticaria may be IgE-mediated or may result from a pharmacological or idiopathic effect. Weals occur as a direct response to chemicals applied directly to the skin. A wide range of substances has been implicated (**Fig. 8.11**). Lesions occur within minutes to hours and resolve in less than 24 hours, leaving normal skin. There is a wide spectrum of clinical presentation in this group, ranging from minor symptoms to an anaphylactic response involving respiratory and gastrointestinal symptoms.

Severe cases of contact urticaria may exhibit both immunological and non-immunological features, and these are of uncertain aetiology. The immunological component is a Type I (IgE-mediated) hypersensitivity reaction, but IgM- and IgG-mediated activations of complement have also been implicated. The non-immunological component, in contrast to that in classical urticaria, is probably prostaglandin-mediated, as severe cases of non-immunological contact urticaria can sometimes be abolished by aspirin or indomethacin.

Substances Implicated as causes of contact urticaria

Chemically defined	Chemically undefined	
Ammonium persulphate	**Animals**	**Textiles**
Bacitracin	Arthropod bites	Wool
Balsam of Peru	Danders	Silk
Benzoic acid	Marine organisms	Rubber
Chloramphenicol	Serum	**Wood**
Chlorpromazine	Saliva	Exotic woods
Epoxy resins	**Cosmetics**	**Foods**
Formaldehyde	Nail varnish	Seafood
Lanolin	Hair spray	Legumes
Para-aminodiphenylamine	Perfume	Nuts
Parabens (ethyl- and methyl-)	**Plants**	Chicken, eggs
Penicillin	Nettles	Flour
Salicylic acid	Cactus	Fruit

Fig. 8.11 Substances implicated as causes of contact urticaria.

Drug-induced urticaria

Acute urticaria is a common manifestation of drug allergy. Aspirin and related non-steroidal anti-inflammatory drugs, penicillins (**Fig. 8.12**) and blood products are the most frequent causes of urticarial drug eruptions, but many other drugs may cause similar symptoms (**Fig. 8.13**). In severe cases, angioedema or a systemic anaphylactic reaction may occur.

symptoms suggesting urticaria

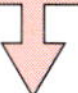

The diagnosis of urticaria is usually self-evident. It may be localized, widespread or florid. The patient complains of swelling with itching. Close observation reveals a shifting pattern of erythema and weals, recently resolved areas being refractory for a few days. Involvement of

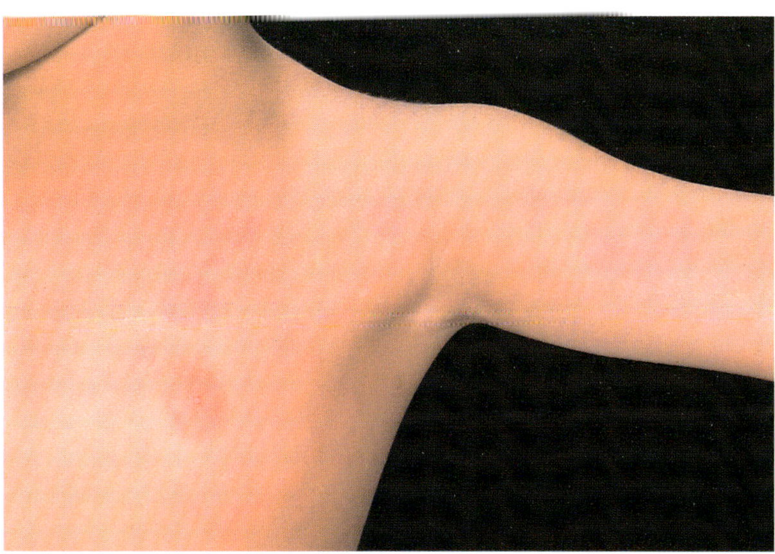

Fig. 8.12 Urticaria following penicillin administration in a young boy.

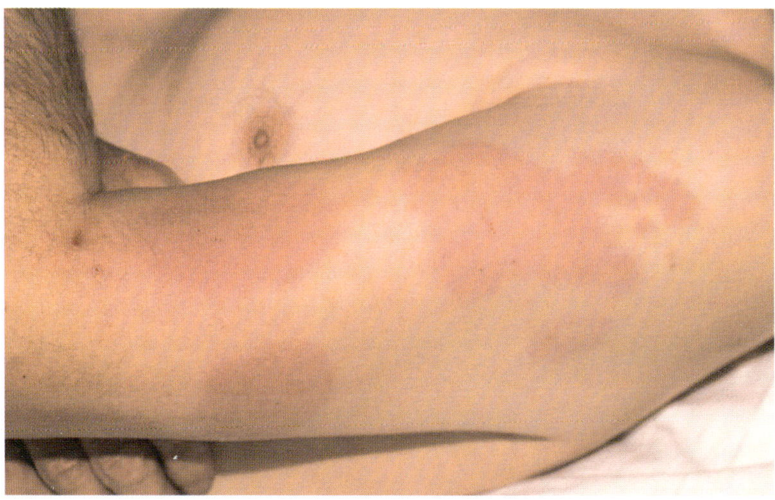

Fig. 8.13 Drug-induced urticaria. Painful pruritic weals developed shortly following subcutaneous injections of heparin in this young man.

mucous membranes and eyelids may be alarming and lesions on the palms and soles may be very painful. Urticaria resolves without trace.

Urticaria induced by contact with allergens or irritants results in redness and weals but can present with burning and stinging. Eczematous lesions, asthma and rhinitis may also occur. The evaluation of the patient to find a cause usually depends on obtaining a thorough history and includes several components (**Fig. 8.14**).

history, examination, and investigation

A photographic record of the patient's appearance during an attack may be helpful (**Fig. 8.15**). A test for dermographism (*see* **Fig. 8.8**) or other physical tests (**Fig. 8.7**) may be useful in confirming the diagnosis of physical urticaria.

After a full history and physical examination, investigations may be planned on the basis of any clues the clinician may have discovered (**Fig. 8.16**).

Acute urticaria

In acute urticaria, a careful, thorough history may reveal an obvious cause. Contact urticaria may be further investigated by direct contact testing with suspected allergens or irritants. Latex rubber has recently been identified as a common and important cause of immunologically mediated contact urticaria. Skin prick tests for Type I hypersensitivity are rarely of value. In atopics, a radioallergosorbent test (RAST) for specific IgE antibodies is sometimes helpful.

Chronic urticaria

For patients with chronic urticaria, a detailed investigation of every possible underlying cause has been shown to be valueless. Where the cause is found, this is usually the result of clues arising from a thorough history and a full examination of the patient.

History and physical examination in urticaria
Location of lesions (generalized, exposed areas, pressure or friction points, sites of exposure to stimulus, etc.)
Morphology of lesions (size, colour, shape, duration)
Pattern of attacks (continuous *versus* intermittent, precipitating factors, associated symptoms)
Review of major types of urticaria
General medical state
Drug history of patient

Fig. 8.14 History and physical examination in urticaria.